PRAISE FOR STROKE STRONG

This book reminded me why stroke recovery is never just medical—it's deeply personal, relational, and life-altering.

As a Physical Medicine & Rehabilitation physician, Erin's honest portrayal of navigating marriage, motherhood, and uncertainty has changed the way I think about the families sitting in front of me in clinic. It's a powerful and generous story.

Alexandra Jensen, DO
Physical Medicine and Rehabilitation Physician

As the Resource Social Worker with the Kentuckiana Stroke Association, I have the privilege of walking alongside stroke survivors and their families every single day. I see the heartbreak, the uncertainty, and the quiet courage it takes to keep moving forward.

This book is not just helpful—it is essential. It will quickly become a staple in the hands of those I serve, because resources that truly meet people in their pain like this are incredibly rare.

This is more than a story. It is a lifeline. And for every person who finds themselves walking through the unthinkable, these pages will remind them they are not alone—and that even here, hope still has a voice.

Dana Robb, Resource Social Worker,
Kentuckiana Stroke Association

As a paramedic, Stroke Outreach Coordinator, and certified Advanced Stroke Coordinator, I have spent years working alongside stroke teams caring for survivors in their most critical moments. But what is often overlooked is the journey that begins after the hospital—the journey carried by the spouse.

This book shines a light on the unsung heroes of stroke recovery: the partners, caregivers, and loved ones who navigate uncertainty, exhaustion, and hope all at once. It is one of the most comprehensive resources available for families, offering both insight and validation for those who stand beside the survivor every step of the way.

If you want to truly understand stroke recovery, you must understand the strength behind the survivor. This book does exactly that.

Brandon Heming, AAS, NRP, ASC-BC
Battalion Chief - Professional Development
Zoneton Fire Protection District

So needed. There is little to guide a survivor, their friends and family and others who want to support them. Unfortunately this story is more common than not. Erin is the most amazing woman who didn't give up no matter how the systems were set up to encourage failure. Brain Injury does not come with an instruction manual and families are often left to "figure" it out on their own.

This family is such an inspiration to others.

Julie Brennan, LSW, CCM,
Marketing Director Caring Moore Homes

As a social worker working with stroke survivors and care-givers daily this book is so eye opening! It's raw, personable, catchy, real and educational. There is so much to learn and teach others. I highly recommend this book!!!

Carrie Crockett, MSSW, CSW,
Stroke Continuum of Care Program Manager at UofL Health

What Erin faced is every spouse's worst fear—watching the person you love slip away while time stands still and moves too fast all at once. In a matter of seconds, her life shifts from ordinary to unimaginable. The fear is raw, the moments are relentless, and the weight of "what if" is crushing.

This is more than the story of a medical emergency—it's a terrifying, deeply human experience of love, helplessness, and strength colliding all at once.

Kevin Moulton, Fire Chief

This book should be handed out with hospital discharge paperwork for any stroke survivor's loved ones, or truly anyone who has suffered a trauma. The author writes through the lens of a caregiver with raw honesty about the stroke experience and aftermath. I finished some chapters with tears in my eyes at the heartbreak… Other times, I found myself giggling and elated at little wins.

It's a candid narrative of the realities of life after trauma and a road map for navigating the aftershocks. I would recommend this book for anyone thrust into the role of caregiver, experiencing a profound life change, or wanting to help someone who is struggling.

Family KY, 5-star Amazon Reviewer

STROKE STRONG

THROUGH THE HEART OF A STROKE SURVIVOR'S WIFE

ERIN TROKLUS

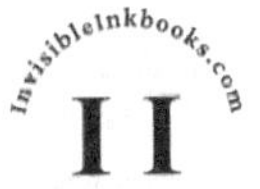

To my husband, Sean—

Thank you for surviving that day and fighting every day since. This life event wasn't in our plans, but we continue to work as a team and fight through it together. I'll always be by your side, no matter what obstacles are thrown our way. Thank you for allowing me to share our story with the world. I love you, for better or worse, for richer or poorer, in sickness and in health, till death do us part.

To my other sisters in the Stroke Survivor's wives club—

None of us wanted to be here, but here we are. We are all stroke strong in our own ways and we're definitely not alone, even on the days we feel that way. May this book provide you with guidance and support. Sending love to you, wherever you may be and wrapping you in hugs and prayers.

One day you will tell your story of how you overcame what you went through and it will be someone else's survival guide.

—Brené Brown

CONTENTS

PART THREE
WE WILL SURVIVE

AUTHOR'S NOTE

This book is written from my memory of my early life and the circumstances that shaped our first year after Sean's stroke. I have done my best to tell the story honestly and accurately, but memory is not perfect—especially when it is shaped by stress, trauma, exhaustion, and the passage of time. Some moments may not be remembered exactly as they happened.

In a few cases, I have shortened timelines or combined events to help the story flow more clearly. Some names and identifying details have been changed to protect privacy. If you remember certain events differently, please know this is simply how I experienced and understood them at the time. Any mistakes are mine alone.

Thank you for reading our story with compassion.

INTRODUCTION

Dear Reader,

I want to share my journey through the first year as a stroke survivor's wife and the events and people that shaped me into the person I am today. My hope is that this provides you with a background on who I am so you will open your heart to my story. If this book finds you facing the unimaginable, you are not alone. I have walked in your shoes and my words may shed some light on questions you haven't had the courage to ask, yet. I started writing this book for me; to process, heal, and track progress. Along the way, I realized others may benefit from a behind the scenes account of going through a life changing event with the one that you love.

While sharing my story in Part One, I provide some help and guidance in navigating the difficult journey of living with and caring for someone during the first year post stroke. Both the challenges you can expect to face and the hope for what could be on the other side of this disability. These are my real and raw personal experiences and the solutions I found helpful as I navigated the dreaded insurance, medical bills, and disability, among many other things. Sorting through your feelings is an ongoing process, but we are often also the ones taking care of the business side. My hope is that, through my experiences of navigating the unknown during the first year, the suggestions outlined in Part Two will now help you with all of those things. And maybe save you a little extra heartache and time in the process. So you can spend that time with your loved one instead.

Part of this story describes the experience of witnessing my husband's stroke and the emotions that followed. These moments can stir strong memories or emotions for those who've walked a similar path. If you, the reader, have experienced a loved one who has had a stroke or other tragic disability, please honor your heart and read at your own pace. Remember, you are not alone in this journey. There are many others out there, going through the same challenges and hardships.

Part Three addresses ways to move forward because it is very easy to feel stuck and overwhelmed. I look at the hard truths of life after a stroke and offer tips and tricks that worked for me. There are many times we are going to feel like it's all too much. Those are the times I want to help you stay *stroke strong*. We have to suit up with every bit of our armor and fight against the stroke that has tried to take us down. We will fight, we will win, and we will survive. One day at a time.

Love,

Erin

PART ONE
MY STORY

My husband, Sean, told me the song "Like Jesus Does" by Eric Church immediately made him think of me when he first heard it in 2011. The fact that he felt my love for him that deeply made me realize I was doing some-thing right as his wife.

When we faced a life-altering event together on a cold, January day in 2025, I wasn't about to let it change his view of me. In fact, I think my love has only grown deeper for him since that day.

Excerpt from "Like Jesus Does"
by Eric Church

All the crazy in my dreams
And both my broken wings
Every single piece of everything I am
And she knows the man I ain't
She forgives me when I can't
The devil, man, no, he don't stand a chance
'Cause she loves me like Jesus does

I always thought she'd give up on me one day
Wash her hands of me, leave me staring down some runway
But I thank God each night and twice on Sunday
That she loves me like Jesus does

CHAPTER 1
NOT YOUR TYPICAL FRIDAY

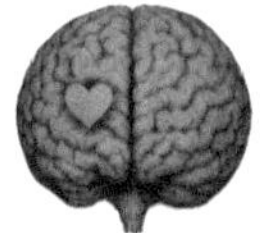

I t was a typical Friday afternoon at the end of a typical week. I had just finished up with my last massage guest for the day, which I was able to move up at the last minute so that my weekend could start a little earlier. I wasn't scheduled to get out of the salon until 5 p.m., so it was a nice surprise when I was able to leave at 4 instead. I texted my husband, Sean, when I pulled out of the parking lot, like I usually do to let him know I was on my way home. I immediately got a response with a thumb's up emoji. We had been texting each other throughout the day between massage guests and meetings. We decided earlier in the day that we'd stay in for dinner that night. Sean worked remotely from home, so he had time to do things around the house and start preparing for dinner. What used to be more of my household duty at the beginning of our marriage had turned into something he started doing and loved.

My commute from the salon was only 20 minutes, so I was pulling in the garage at 4:20 p.m. I gathered my items and walked into the house from the garage door. I passed our bedroom door to lay my purse on the hope chest at the entrance to our kitchen. I glanced at the kitchen bar and sure enough, Sean had already started prepping dinner. The veggies were cut and placed in individual containers and the chicken was seasoned and laid out waiting for me to arrive home before he started to cook. I turned around to walk in the bedroom. Sean was coming out of our ensuite bathroom.

"Hey babe," I greeted him. He was walking unusually sluggish and dragging his right side along with him. His head was down.

"What are you doing?" I asked. Confused and even a little amused, thinking he was messing with me, imitating a scene from *The Walking Dead*. He slowly pulled his head up, as if it weighed a hundred pounds. That's when I immediately noticed that the right side of his face was completely drooping.

"Oh my gosh! Do I need to call 9-1-1? When did this start?" Only mumbles and sounds came out. No words. Without hesitation, I dialed the number that no one wants to ever have to call.

"9-1-1, what's your emergency?" The voice on the other end of the line was calm and collected.

I, on the other hand, was anything but calm. My voice was shaky, and I spoke with sheer panic. "I think my husband is having a stroke!"

The moments that followed were somewhat of a blur. I remember answering all the operator's questions – address, health history, medications, and the signs and symptoms he was showing right before my very eyes. But I was also keeping an eye on Sean during the question-and-answer session. He had managed to drag himself over to the edge of the bed. One side was on the bed, while the other was sliding off. I was growing more impatient with the operator and felt the anxiety growing at an exponential rate.

"If anything changes before EMS arrives, give us a call back." I threw my phone down and went over to Sean.

You hear stories of how people almost leave their body when there is tragedy and the adrenaline kicks in. That's exactly what I did. My super-human strength kicked in and I successfully got a 180-pound body on the floor. I just kept thinking how I needed to get him off the bed and laying down, so he didn't fall.

My voice remained shaky, but now I was screaming. "Sean, Sean, SEAN, SEAN!! Stay with me. Help is on the way!" I, too, was on the floor crouching over his almost limp body and was cupping the back of his neck so his head wouldn't hit the floor. He was increasingly becoming heavier as the minutes and seconds passed.

Now, I started the question-and-answer session with him. "Are you hurting anywhere?! Can you breathe okay?! Are you having any chest pains?!" I was barely even giving him enough time to answer me. And when he tried, the once-unrecognizable mumbles had turned into grunts only. There was now no attempt to formulate words. Or should I say, he couldn't formulate words. Then, his eyes started to roll back and I was losing him.

"If anything changes, call us back." The words from the operator echoed back to me. I called 9-1-1 back. I was now alternating screaming with fear at the operator and then back to Sean, trying to hold the phone up to my ear while holding Sean's head. I no longer could keep the tears from falling. I had officially let fear take over and my screams turned into a pleading cry.

"Ma'am, they are on route and should be there soon." But soon wasn't soon enough. I needed them to be here *now*. Sean was slipping into unconsciousness, and I just *knew* if I let him close his eyes, he'd be gone forever. I continued to beg him to stay with me and resorted to smacking his face. Every time I'd yell his name, his eyes would temporarily pop back open which would only be followed up by closing again. I was running out of time.

In the midst of all the chaos, I forgot that our son, Austin, was home. Being a typical 15-year-old, he had returned home from school an hour before and crashed in his room, door closed, headphones on, deep into a video game with his friends. And it didn't help that his bedroom was on the other side of the house. He had no idea what was going on with his dad, mere feet away on the other side of his bedroom door. I yelled for him as loud as I could from our bedroom floor. I didn't want to leave Sean, but I knew I needed Austin's help. By some miracle that could have only been God's intervention, Austin heard me. He came running out of this room and stood in our doorway.

He was quickly updated from the scene that I can only imagine is ingrained into his head forever.

"Dad is having a stroke. The ambulance is on their way and I need you to watch out for them!" He stepped up, no questions asked. He ran down to the end of our driveway to be on the lookout and wave the emergency crews in when they arrived.

WHEN would they arrive? It felt like it had been hours since I made the call, but realistically it had been around fifteen minutes. Still, fifteen minutes was too long. *Now what do I do? Just wait? I can't just wait! Time is too precious,* and I didn't have the time. Or should I say, Sean didn't have the time. *Should I call 9-1-1 back again?*

Ricky. That's who I'll call. Ricky is Sean's best friend, but they refer to each other as brothers. They grew up together and lived with one another throughout their childhood and as young adults. Ricky has been in my life from the time I met Sean and was the Best Man in our wedding. Ricky was also an ER nurse for over ten years. *He'll know what to do, right?* I called Ricky and thankfully, he immediately answered. His cheerful "hello" quickly turned to emergent Nurse Ricky mode when I told him what was going on. By that point, I was in a full cry, had every unimaginable thought running through my head, and Sean's grunts had become no noise at all. His mouth would open and absolutely nothing came out. Silence. His eyes were staying shut even longer in between my face slaps and yelling his name.

I managed to fumble through my phone and called Ricky back on Facetime because he wanted to see Sean. After all, he couldn't decipher much and make his medical evaluation with just me talking – more blubbering – at him. Within a couple minutes of Ricky's phone evaluation, the garage door swung open, and in ran Austin. Behind him, was a large, bearded man maybe in his early 30s. He rolled in with confidence and a take-charge attitude. And behind him, was a whole crew. It was 4:45 p.m. For the first time in 24 minutes, I felt myself take a breath. Help had arrived.

I stepped away and let the professionals get to work saving my husband. By this point, Sean wasn't opening his eyes at all. I watched from afar, tears still stinging my eyes and silently saying another prayer. I saw everyone stepping in like an assembly line, working in unison. IVs were getting started, the blood pressure cuff put on, stickers being tossed on the floor frantically so that heart monitor pads could be put on his chest. It was organized chaos.

The in-charge man took me to the side. "Can you write your husband's name, social security number and date of birth down for me?" Although I realized he probably really did need this information, I think it was also a clever tactic to get me out of the room. I went into the kitchen and found a piece of scrap paper in the junk drawer. I scribbled "Sean Troklus, his social, and DOB December 1980" and gave it to Mr. In-Charge. Yes, Sean was a newly 44 year-old and he was having a stroke. Austin was standing in the kitchen in silence. He didn't know what to say. He probably wanted to cry but was trying to be strong. After all, I was a big enough mess for both of us.

I heard Ricky's voice. I realized, in the chaos, I never hung up the phone with him and he was still on the other end of the line, listening to everything going on.

"Where are they taking him?" he asked. I could tell he was already on the road and still in nurse mode. Panicked too, but remaining calm. Mr. In-Charge said they were taking him to the closest hospital to us, just five minutes down the road and in our county. It wasn't Ricky's first choice, as he felt Sean needed to go to a hospital that could do emergent surgery, if God forbid, that would be necessary. But everywhere else was too far away and I knew we had already wasted so much time. I saw how fast I was losing Sean. I wasn't going to risk that. So, against Ricky's judgement, my take-charge attitude came out in conjunction with my adrenaline and made the executive decision to go to our county hospital. Ironically, Ricky and I both used to work there, so he had already reached out to all his connections to let them know that Sean was heading their direction.

It took no time for them to have Sean loaded on a gurney and in the back of the ambulance. Due to the emergent care he was requiring, I was unable to ride with him. I had to follow behind. Austin and I jumped in my car in the garage and waited for the ambulance to pull out so we could follow them. I was shaking from head to toe, my heart was pounding, and my head was spinning. Out of nowhere, Ricky showed up at my car door window. He knew I was breaking down and he had to take over.

"You're not driving right now, it's not safe" he instructed. "Get out, I'm driving you." Even though I didn't want to move, I knew he was right. I was in no position or head space to be driving, even if it was just 5 minutes down the road. We managed to somehow arrive at the ER before the ambulance even arrived. Just like Ricky said, the staff knew we were coming and were waiting for us on our arrival.

We weren't there 3 minutes when we heard over the deafening loud intercom system "Code Stroke, Emergency Room. Code Stroke, Emergency Room. Code Stroke, Emergency Room." My stomach turned and I physically thought I was going to get sick. I waited impatiently in one of the waiting room chairs. Austin sat in silence across the room from me, holding on to Sean's wallet and phone. Ricky stood up at the ER reception desk, chatting with the security guard that was on duty that night.

I sat there in my thoughts and knew I was going to need to call Sean's parents. Mike and Karen had been residing at their lake house for the last five years in Columbia, Kentucky so they were almost a 2-hour drive away. If this was as bad as I thought it might be, I needed to go ahead and let them know. I dialed Karen's number and dreaded her picking up the phone. I don't think I got the full sentence out before I was in tears again. She managed to finally understand me and said they would get on the road and keep them updated with any changes. I got off the phone, dried up my tears and headed over to sit next to Austin. I knew I had to get into mom mode and check on my son. He had just been through a lot. He is a smart kid, mature for his age so I knew he recognized the severity of the situation.

I looked at him and asked, "Do you think I should go ahead and call Landon?" Landon is our 19-year-old son. He was in his sophomore year at Eastern Kentucky University, and he had just arrived in Gatlinburg, Tennessee for a formal with his fraternity. In fact, while we were sitting in the waiting room, Sean's phone buzzed. It was Landon sending him a picture of the views from their mountain chalet of the Smokey Mountains letting him know they arrived safely. He had been so excited for this trip. I didn't want to worry him unnecessarily, but I also knew he would be mad if I didn't let him know what was going on.

Austin looked at me with worried eyes, but said in the most caring voice, "Just wait Mom. Let's see what is going on and then you can call him."

"Are you okay?" I asked him.

"Yeah, I'm fine." I knew he was trying to put on a brave face. We sat there for what seemed like forever, then the doctor came and escorted us to "the family room." I knew we weren't about to get good news. You don't get taken to a family room when there's good news. Only bad.

Sure enough, the doctor sat the three of us down and with a solemn expression, said "The CT showed a large brain bleed on the left side of his brain in the basal ganglia area, which caused Sean to have a hemorrhagic stroke. His blood pressure is 250/170. We've had to intubate him. He has been given blood pressure medications to stabilize him and we've had to sedate him with Versed, Fentanyl and…" The doctor's voice started trailing off.

I could see his mouth moving, but comprehending everything he was saying was almost impossible.

He continued, "We are going to need to transfer him downtown to University of Louisville Hospital." Now I knew that wasn't good. U of L is the hospital you go to for trauma. It wasn't a hospital you wanted to visit someone in or be the patient in. In fact, my body went hot and I immediately had a flashback and PTSD of the last time I was in U of L Hospital.

It was in April 2000. I was dating Chris, and we were pretty serious at the time. He had been on his way to my house when he crashed his truck into a tree. He had to be stat-flighted to, yep, you guessed it, U of L hospital. He hit his head on impact with the tree which caused his brain to swell. After a week in a coma in the ICU, Chris passed away. That experience still haunts me. I remember every detail, including holding his mom's hand, promising her that we would remain in each other's lives from that moment on. After all, Chris was Kathy's only child.

That was my personal experience at U of L Hospital. *And they were going to take my husband there!? I'd be damned if I was going to go through that again. I couldn't go through that again.*

I zoned back in to the doctor who was still speaking and then asked in a concerned voice, "Do you have any questions for me?"

Ricky chimed in with questions of his own, several that I didn't understand as he started speaking in medical jargon. I was so thankful to have him there to comprehend the things I couldn't, but it's also a double-edged sword when you know too much about the diseases, disabilities, and pathologies that are out there. As an ER nurse, he had seen things. He knew how bad things could get. I could see Ricky was fighting his own struggle with this. Knowing the severity and coming from a medical point of view, but also knowing Sean is his best friend, not just a stranger patient, that we were talking about.

Landon. I had to ask what I should do about Landon. "Excuse me, but do you think I need to call my son who is away at college?" I knew what the doctor's answer was going to be, but there was a part of me just hoping he was going to tell me no.

With a grim look, he answered, "I can't tell you what you should do, but if it were me, I'd have him come in as soon as possible." There it is again. The stinging in my eyes. He concluded with "You can go back and see him, if you'd like, before we transfer him downtown."

Ricky and I walked down the empty halls to the transfer room they had Sean in. Austin chose not to go back and see Sean there, and I wasn't going to pressure him to do so. His 15-year-old brain had just taken in a lot of adult information. I knew he just needed to process it all in his own way. When we walked around the corner into the room, it was a sight I'll never forget. Sean was completely unconscious. His clothes had been cut off and he was in one of those dingy blue hospital gowns. Every piece of equipment in that room was hooked up to him. There were tubes and IVs and monitors attached to what looked like every inch of his body. A nurse came in and handed me a bag with his shoes and belongings in it. I forced a "thank you" but couldn't take my eyes off of Sean.

I went over and grabbed his hand, kissed him on the forehead, and whispered "I love you" in his ear. In a matter of two hours, our lives just turned upside down. This was anything but a typical Friday.

CHAPTER 2

EVERYTHING HAPPENS FOR A REASON

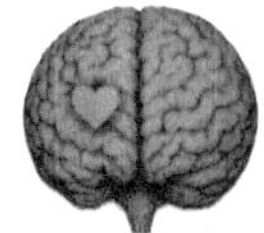

try not to question God when things happen in life, but the human side of me finds that hard to do at times, especially when those things are tragedies. Over time, I've adopted the saying "Everything Happens for a Reason." Yes, it's cliché and even cringe to some, but it has helped me make sense of the bad things in life. My personality requires explanations and the answer to my "whys." And I don't necessarily require immediate answers to those events. In fact, I've found that the majority of the time, I don't get an answer until months, or sometimes years, afterwards.

I met Chris through mutual friends who set us up on a blind date. I was hesitant about going out with someone that I had never met, but I trusted my friends. The conversation with Chris was easy from the beginning and the physical chemistry was there immediately. The first date turned into a second one just two days later, which then turned into daily late-night conversations that would last for hours. We felt very comfortable with one another from day one, therefore a few months of knowing one another felt like years. Our feelings were strong and moved fast and we were in love within a short period of time. At that moment, I truly thought Chris may have been "the one." So when he died tragically from a car accident at the age of 21, this was difficult to understand. Why would God rob someone of their life at such a young age? Why would he take away Kathy's only child? Chris was someone that I thought, at the time, was my forever person, so that heartbreaking loss was excruciatingly painful to my young heart.

Fast forward a year to when I met Sean. Sean and Chris shared a lot of the same personality traits. They were both funny and always the life of the party, but they each had kind and sentimental sides too. At first, I was very nervous to open my heart to Sean, scared that he would be taken away from me, too. But, as time went on, I was able to let go of that fear, I opened up and let Sean in. He made that easy to do and was extremely understanding of my past with Chris and the fears that went along with the tragedy. His understanding and love made me quickly fall hard for him and I knew within no time that I was meant to be with Sean. So "Everything Happens for a Reason" proved true and Sean was actually my person, not Chris. But that didn't explain why Chris had to lose his life. I could have still ended up with Sean while Chris got to live.

My relationship with my own mother became very toxic starting in middle school and only got worse as the years passed. There was a short period of time, when I was in 9th grade, when she separated from my dad for a few months. She was a stay-at-home mom at the time, so my dad paid for her to move into her own furnished apartment to figure out her feelings and decide what she wanted. I was crushed, left at home to help my dad with my three younger sisters, who were between the ages of 8 and 13 years old at the time. Being the oldest, I felt a responsibility to my family to take the place my mom left behind. With my dad working outside the house full-time, someone had to be at home with them during the day. I helped with fixing their hair, assigning them chores, entertaining them, and preparing dinners. My sisters probably viewed me as bossy and irritating, but I was just doing what I thought was right at the time. I was hurting and confused too, but I didn't have time to show it. I was cursed with being the oldest, therefore I took on the responsibilities that go along with holding that position in the family. My sole purpose at that time was to be there for my dad and help raise my sisters. All while my mom chose to live her own life in her own apartment, without her family.

I know I was young at the time and I probably couldn't fully grasp the magnitude of the adult situation that was taking place, but I do know how the events affected me personally. It's still a time in my life that is hard to wrap my head around. The separation lasted for about four months, then my mom decided to return home. I'd like to tell you that she figured out her feelings and things got better when she came home but things were anything but good. It was awkward, and full of tension and resentment. I felt like she wanted to pick up where she left off before moving out and start being a mom again without noticing I had been the mom for several months. That didn't settle well with me. I started talking back and being defiant to her, which I had never done before. I simply wanted to hurt her like she hurt me.

I distinctly remember a time, just days after she had returned home, she told me to do my laundry. I looked at her and without hesitation, blatantly said "No." Then followed up with, "If Daddy asks me to do laundry, then I'll do it." I knew that comment would be a jab to her, but I didn't care. I was trying to make a point. And did it ever. My mother demanded respect and I refused to give it to her. We proceeded to get madder and louder as we took the argument into my parent's room. My dad came in to try and deescalate the matter.

"What are you going to do, spank me?" And with that comment, I turned my outer thigh over and pointed, basically daring her to do something. With that, she hauled off and slugged me across the cheek. I was in such shock that I just froze. My sisters and I all had our fair share of spankings, but we were never hit in the face. But there I was, sitting in disbelief and my cheek stinging with the aftermath of the hit. At that point, I just lost it. I don't know what was louder, my screaming or my crying. My dad quickly intervened and proceeded to escort my mom out of the room to separate us. I just couldn't bear the pain I felt that was caused from her decisions.

I got a little braver each day and began telling her how hurt I felt when she made the decision to leave.That didn't settle well within our formerly close mother-daughter relationship. My dad was who I leaned on now, not my mom. I would only take direction from him, not her. I respected him, not her. The once healthy relationship was turning toxic. She was like a bowl of ice cream; something I craved, but wasn't healthy to consume. I felt like her heart just wasn't into being a mother and I could see she had fallen out of love with my dad.

The night before my second semester in college, I got a call from my dad. My mom had officially left. She had packed up her things and moved in permanently with a friend. He broke the news to me through tears. I could hear the devastation in my dad's voice. He felt like he failed us girls. But I saw a man who fought for his family until he couldn't fight any longer. He was worn down and in immense pain. I was hurt too, but wasn't surprised by the news. After I completed that semester, I chose to stop my college career and return home to work and help my dad full time. It wasn't what I had planned for my life, but it was an easy decision at the time. My priority was my dad and sisters, not my future.

Time and time again, my mom and I continued to clash over life decisions. At first, I forgave her and gave her multiple chances to make things right. After all, I craved that bowl of ice cream. But after decades of pain and trying to move on a number of times, I came to the conclusion it just wasn't feasible to have a healthy relationship with my own mom. I was the only one that continued to be hurt and I finally had enough. I finally chose to do what was best for myself. I also wasn't going to allow my own children to go through that same pain. So, in my mid-30s, I officially broke off contact with my mom and we became estranged. At that time, it was both the easiest and most difficult decision I ever had to make. But having a painful relationship with my mom was another thing in my life that made me question "why?"

After Chris passed, it only made sense for Kathy and I to become close. We both yearned for a relationship that we were missing in our lives. So, I kept my promise to her and she is an important part of my life, even to this day. I am still so grateful that Sean not only accepted my relationship with Kathy and the unusual situation but also embraced her in his life as well. Over the years, she has been an unwavering part of our family. She has been there for me, Sean, and our boys more times than I can even count. She has attended Christmases, birthdays, baptisms and graduations. She slowly moved into the role as another grandmother to the boys, attending Grandparent's Days at their schools, ball games, and drumming gigs. And she became my mom.

On a cold November day, years after Chris' passing and years after my break up with my mom, Kathy and I were out for our yearly Christmas shopping trip. It is a day we look forward to every year. We were shopping and chatting as usual, and it hit us like a ton of bricks. She was a mother without a child, and I was a child without a mother. We were always meant to be in one another's lives! It was finally the answer we both had been searching for as to the why of such tragic and heartbreaking events. Everything happens for a reason.

Then there was the loss of my dad in 2014 when he was just 62 years old. In my opinion, he was still young. He had a massive heart attack and three days later, after never leaving the hospital, passed away. Another tragic heartbreak. I was extremely close to my dad, your typical "Daddy's Girl." He was the rock in my life. My dad was the most unselfish, loving, God-fearing man. I have so many fond memories of him as a child. Although he worked full time, he was a very hands-on dad. He'd come home exhausted from work, I'm sure, but hardly ever said "no" to his girls when we wanted to spend time with him. We'd go in the yard to throw a ball or hike the trails in the woods behind our home. We'd pick blackberries and he taught us how to eat honeysuckles. Slowly pulling out the center part of the flower and eating the sweet honey-like sap that was extracted from the plant. I still can't pass that sweet smell of honeysuckle without thinking of him.

As I got a little older, I'd anticipate his arrival home from work and would run down to the end of our street to meet him as he pulled into our cul-de-sac. I'd see that blue, hatchback Honda pull around the corner and he'd always stop to let me in the car. I'd jump in, hop in his lap on the driver's side and he'd let me "drive" the rest of the way to our house. Those small things were so big to me. His love for his kids was also matched with discipline when we needed it. The worst thing ever was disappointing my dad. So, even though we'd get the occasional smack on the leg for misbehaving, the words "you've disappointed me" were worse than any spanking or punishment I'd ever received. As I entered my teen years, no doubt becoming a more difficult kid, I heard those words a little more.

Lying was a big thing for him. It took just one time of me lying to my dad about where I was for the night, and I never did that again. To this day, I don't lie in fear that I'll still get a talking to from my dad from beyond the grave. We'd always dread the "Daddy lectures," as we called them. Not only because they seemed to last forever (he really had a knack for going on and on and on), but the maddening way that he would never yell. He would say everything in a calm and collected tone, talking slowly and with intent. As a child, it was torture and would not end fast enough. And he'd always finish the lectures with "I love you" and a hug. He was pretty good at making you feel the guilt of your bad decisions. But despite that, I never once doubted his love for myself or my sisters, and in the future, Sean and his grandchildren.

As we grew into adults, his lectures became sound advice and I valued his opinion on any obstacle life threw my way. It always came from a place of love and non-judgement. With four daughters, there was rarely a time when he wasn't mending a disagreement between us. When he had his heart attack we were all devastated. His passing proved that he was the glue that was holding the family together. We all knew then, but it was even more evident after the fact. Again, I questioned "why?" It was unfortunate and sad that over time, the family relationships started to crumble.

During the times my dad would have stepped in to mend relationships, talk sense into us, or give us Godly advice, he wasn't there. And the consequences of that spoke volumes. I tried to step up and take on that responsibility of holding relationships with my sisters together. I had a few successes but ended up failing miserably. I grieved those broken relationships and although it still hurts to this day, I've learned to cope with that and move on. As much as it hurts to lose people, especially my family, that were once such a huge part of my life, I know it would have destroyed my dad. He was bound to die from a broken heart one way or another and God chose to take him early to spare him from the heartbreak of his own children not talking to one another. Everything Happens for a Reason.

Now, here I am, trying to make sense of why Sean had a stroke at 44 years old. What's the reason? Maybe it's a way to strengthen our relationship? Maybe it's to be a poster child of Men's Health? That it's never too early to get regular check-ups at the doctor and exercise and take care of the one body that you are given. His tag line could even be, "Don't be a stubborn ass like me and get your check-ups." Okay, so maybe that's a little extreme, but it's a start. Remember, I'm still trying to make sense of this situation. Or maybe there will be doors that open up in his future that never would have even been there unless he had this stroke. I don't know the reason right now. But just like all the other tragic things in my past, I have no doubt that I will know the reason for this event too. It's just a matter of when.

CHAPTER 3
LUCK OF THE IRISH

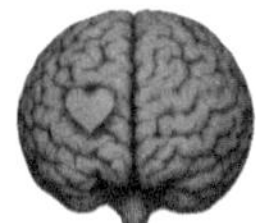

I t was St. Patrick's Day 2001. The Shaggy song "It Wasn't Me" was blasting out of Amanda's black Toyota 4Runner. It was a Saturday night and everyone was going out. We cruised down Bardstown Road in the Highlands, an area of town in Louisville that was known for the best bars and nightclubs. We landed at a local Irish Pub, which was the perfect place to start the night. The bar was packed with people with the sounds of Irish music playing and pints of green beer being chugged all around us. St. Patrick's celebrations have always been big in Louisville, with a huge parade and block party a few weeks leading up to the day and parties everywhere during the weekend. That year was no exception, and the weather was particularly nice so everyone showed up in droves.

Amanda and I hung out there for a bit before we headed down a few blocks to Have a Nice Day Café. The club was known for classic 70s and 80s music. The kind of music where everyone knew every word, especially the girl anthems like "Respect" by Aretha Franklin or "Summer Lovin'" from the Grease soundtrack. Later in the night, the DJ would throw in crude songs like Def Leppard's "Pour Some Sugar on Me" or George Michael's "I Want Your Sex."

That really got the crowd going. And everyone would be dancing. Everyone. A few guys might linger around the bar waiting to buy a drink for the next girl who walked up, but everyone else would be on the dance floor. It was the spot to be.

We went every weekend, and we weren't about to skip out on one of the biggest party weekends of the year. The line to get in wrapped all the way around the building, but it was always worth the wait. As we approached the door the sounds of the classic tunes were blaring out the entrance. We showed our IDs to the bouncer and went straight to the bar. I got my usual at the time, cranberry and vodka while Amanda got her Miller Lite. We headed to the dance floor to join up with the rest of the bar. The floor was sticky from the sugary drinks spilled from the party goers the night before. Wall to wall 20-somethings, with your occasional underage drinkers, filled the club. The smell of alcohol, sweat, cigarettes, cologne, and puke filled the air and it was fantastic in every way.

Attached to Have a Nice Day Café, connected by a door walkway, was Bar Louisville. Although just as packed, the vibe was very different there. The smells were all the same but the music was different. They played the current pop music mixed with what we now call "Old School" Rap. A large square bar was directly in the middle of the club, where you not only got your next drink, but the girls would get on top of it and dance around while the guys gawked from below. It was trashy for sure, but the most fun. I was guilty a time or two of getting up there with all my girls. I opted out of the bar dancing that night though.

"Erin!," I faintly heard someone screaming my name from across the club. Amanda was dancing next to me so I knew it wasn't her. It was my long time friend, Ali, who I hadn't seen in a few years. We hugged and caught up, screaming through the loud music and pushing our way through the crowd to get over to the side to try and remotely even hear one another.

She screamed, "Hey, are you single?!" It had been 11 months since Chris had passed away and I was open to start dating again but just hadn't met anyone that sparked my interest.

"Yeah, I'm single. Why?"

"Hey Sean!" she screamed again to a guy across the way. *What in the world was she doing?* "Erin, this is Sean. Sean, this is Erin. Bye!" And just like that, she smiled and darted away.

What is happening here? All I knew was I had lost Amanda in the process of running into Ali and now she left me with this guy I didn't know. *But this guy. Man, was he hot. But I couldn't let him know I thought he was hot.* The song "Butterfly" by Crazy Town started playing.

"Wanna dance?" he asked, screaming over the music.

HELL YEAH, I thought. But instead settled for the subtle, "okay." We started dancing and wouldn't you know, that not only was he hot, but he could dance too. Yikes, I was in trouble. The smiles grew on our faces, and we got closer and closer to one another while we danced. *Did he think I was hot too?* No way, I couldn't be that lucky.

He leaned in to kiss me, but I put my finger up to his lips confidently stating "what kind of a girl do you think I am?" Although my gut was saying *kiss him you idiot,* I decided to go for the play-hard-to-get route and just hope it would work to my benefit. And lucky for me, it did. We ended up dancing together the rest of the night, closing down the place at 4 a.m. when the music faded and the lights came on.

He walked me and Amanda back to her 4Runner. Our voices were hoarse from the yelling and the smells of the bar were now all over our clothes and hair.

"What are you doing tomorrow?" he asked.

"Going to church." I answered, with a somewhat evil flirtatious grin. I didn't know if the devil or angel side of me was coming out.

"Why don't you and Amanda meet me and my friend afterwards at the park to go 4-wheeling?" I had never been 4-wheeling, but I knew I wanted to see Sean again, so I was willing to meet him wherever and do whatever to see him again. We agreed on a place and time to meet them the next afternoon. I went home that night feeling pretty good about myself. The luck of the Irish was definitely on my side that evening. I was giddy with excitement and couldn't wait to meet him the following day.

The next day, I went to church with my dad like the good girl that I was, quickly changed clothes and left to meet up with Amanda, Sean and his friend. We met at a gas station near the park. When we pulled in, there he was leaning up against a bright red F-150 with his ball cap on backwards and filling up his 4-wheeler with gas. *Oh. My. Gosh. Who was this guy?* I never met anyone like him before, but the butterflies in my stomach were telling me this could be a good thing.

We got to the park and unloaded the 4-wheelers. He gave me a helmet and I innocently played helpless like I had no idea what I was doing. Which to be honest, I kind of didn't, so I was able to play that to my advantage. I hopped on the back of the 4-wheeler and away we went. He made sure to drive fast and go through every mud puddle and sharp curve he could find. Showing off no doubt, so if he was doing it just to impress me, it was working. We stopped in a clearing in the woods. We had lost Amanda and his friend along the way somewhere so it was just us. We took our helmets off and took a breather. I flirtatiously complained about the scrapes on my leg from the tree branches hitting them going through the trails and he flirtatiously apologized.

Then it happened. He leaned in to kiss me and this time I did not play hard to get. I let him. And you guessed it. This hot dancer that drove a big truck was also a great kisser. I felt like a cartoon character, where the googly eyes were popping out of my head and my heart was pumping out of my chest. That kiss was totally worth the wait, and we both knew it.

We continued seeing one another regularly after that day. He worked the night shift and I was on days so timing could be tricky, but we still managed to make time. It was only weeks after St. Patrick's Day that we were introducing one another to each other's parents and families and friends. Ironically, since we went to high schools down the road from one another, we actually had a lot of friends in common. The odds of us never meeting before that night was pretty crazy actually as we realized we had even been at the same parties. But it just goes to show you that timing is everything. Things moved quickly and within 2 months, Sean told me he loved me. I had a feeling it was coming soon, and I was nervous about it. I didn't know for sure if I was ready for "love." But when he said it, my reflex immediately said it back. And what was once making me nervous, felt so right. I did love this man.

Sean proposed to me in July 2002 on a beach in the Bahamas. We were on a couple's trip with my best friend, Jill, and her boyfriend. They were in on the plan and helped smuggle the engagement ring on the plane. I left on the trip with a boyfriend and came home with a fiancé. We were so happy and in love. I really didn't think I could feel this way about someone else. Our engagement lasted a little over a year and in October 2003, we got married. It was the happiest day of my life. Our song we danced to at our wedding reception was "My Best Friend" by Tim McGraw. It was a song that Sean picked out for us just months into our relationship. He was big into music and lyrics and he said the song was "just perfect" for us. And it really was. Who would have thought that a guy I met through a friend at a bar would become my husband and best friend? We still thank Ali every year on St. Patrick's Day and our wedding anniversary for her match-making skills.

Our first year of marriage was truly like a honeymoon. We very rarely argued and just enjoyed building a life together. Things continued to move along perfectly. The mention of a baby started to come up in conversation. We were still young, but I was ready. Sean wanted to stew on the idea a little longer. But after holding our nephew, Michael, in the hospital after he was born he came home that night and told me he was ready to start trying. We were in the process of building a house, but figured since it would probably take a while to get pregnant, we'd go ahead and get the ball rolling. Three months later, on the weekend we moved into our new home, I found out I was pregnant. We were shocked but over-the-moon excited. We welcomed Landon into the world in September 2005.

Navigating parenthood had its normal challenges, but it was even harder because I felt like a single parent during the majority of the week. I could feel Sean crawl in the bed and let out a sigh from his long night working on the assembly line. I could make out the smell of a fresh shower and deodorant that still had the strong aroma of just being applied. He would cuddle up next to me and wrap his arms around me. My eyes peeled open to look at the alarm clock. It was always around 4 a.m. I had about 90 minutes in the bed with him before my alarm would go off. I was so very tired.

Training a newborn to sleep through the night and be up during the day poses challenges for any new parent, but even more so when Sean and I worked opposite shifts. Our own days and nights were mixed up so how were we supposed to sleep train a baby? I managed to figure it out but that also meant I was the only one to get up every time Landon would cry. So my sleep was broken up every night for about ten months.

It felt like I was only back to sleep for 5 minutes and my alarm would go off. By that point, Sean was deep into his sleep and more than likely, snoring. I got up, threw myself together and was at work by 6:30 a.m. My work day was pretty mundane and for the most part just going through the motions. Meanwhile, Sean was going on about 3 hours of sleep before Landon would wake up for the day. He too, was so very tired, trying to sleep whenever Landon would nap during the day. He'd start getting ready for his work day around the same time I'd wrap up my shift. I'd get home to be greeted by Sean and Landon waiting for me in the garage.

"Have a great day," I said to Sean.

"Have a great night," he'd say back to me, almost in unison. And with a kiss and a quick 'I love you,' Landon would be transferred from Sean's arms and into mine and we'd wave good-bye as he pulled out of the drive. We were like two ships sailing in the night, except we felt more like robots and probably looked more like zombies. But it was wonderfully exhausting.

Sean was an amazing, loving father and we soaked up every moment of parenthood. Luckily, we had the same views when it came to raising children. We agreed on how we would discipline, how we would handle different hurdles along the way, and how we would celebrate milestones and we've held true to those beliefs over the years.

Things were moving along with our happy family of 3, but Sean and I both were starting to be unhappy with our jobs. I had been working in administrative assistant and secretary-type jobs and I just wasn't happy. I was good at what I did, but I wasn't being fulfilled. I felt limited on what I could do though. I had a 2-year-old at home and only 40 college credits under my belt. It would take forever to go back to school to get my degree as I had to continue to work full time. I had been working in a hospital setting for about seven years. I loved the idea of helping people, but knew that nursing wasn't my calling. After researching around and with Sean's support, I decided to attend massage therapy school.

It was a career path I was always interested in but never really thought I'd pursue. I signed up and was committed to school for two years, figuring *I can do anything for two years, right?* Looking back, I honestly have no idea how we did it. My alarm went off every morning at 4:30 a.m., which meant the 90 minutes we once had with one another daily, decreased to 30 minutes. I sluggishly and slowly peeled myself out of the bed every morning. The sun hadn't started to rise when I arrived at work around 5:30 a.m. It would still be night shift when I'd clock in every morning. Since no one else in my department had arrived yet, it would be an opportunity to get a lot of work done without distractions. But the silence in the office also made it hard to keep my eyes open at times. Three hours of work would be followed up by a 30 minute commute to massage school, where I'd be for the next 3 hours, then back to work to finish the rest of my shift. By 3:30 p.m. I was headed home for the Landon hand off.

I ended up graduating valedictorian of my class and started my massage career within 2 months of receiving my massage therapy license. I filled in for another therapist at a local salon and spa. It was temporary work. I had no desire to work in a spa setting. I felt all my education would go to waste and planned to pursue a job in a more medical setting. I was proven wrong within a short period of time working in the salon. I loved my boss and I really connected with the guests. I learned quickly that it wasn't just pampering services and playing with fun aromas. People really wanted to be helped with their ailments and pains, and I was the one helping them. I was able to use what I learned in school and educate them on the importance of massage therapy for not just the body, but the mind. I looked forward to seeing guests return to me over and over and they enjoyed the hour spent with me. I've connected with them on so many levels, not just as a therapist in their self care, but as a friend. It was exactly the career fulfillment that I had been searching for.

Shortly after I graduated massage school and got licensed, Sean started talking about a career move for him. He always said that he wasn't going to stay on night shift once Landon started in sports and school. He didn't want to miss out on being a coach or attending school events. When his company offered early buy-outs in 2008, he decided to take the plunge and leave the assembly line job he knew for the last nine years to work as a mortgage broker. He had been training under a friend for several months and built his confidence to make the career change. Plus, the buy-out allowed us to pay off our car and my school loan.

We were trying to make big changes in our lives and be as respon-sible as possible about it along the way. It wasn't easy, but we wanted to prove to everyone that we could do it. We were capable of creating this life that we dreamed of. Were these decisions scary financially? Yes. Were we ever afraid that maybe we were making life-changing decisions too soon? Yes. But our relationship was strong and we always did a really good job at openly communi-cating with one another. If one of us was unsure or hesitant, we were comfortable enough to talk it over with one another. Mutual respect in our relationship was a value we prided ourselves on.

Throughout the first several years of marriage, we managed to find our groove and responsibilities within our relationship, while also embracing our roles as parents. We utilized one another's strengths to make the household run smoothly. I used my analyt-ical and organizational strengths by handling the finances, laun-dry, appointments, and schedules for the family. Sean used his creative strengths by taking care of the house, yard, and vehicles, and over time started taking over the cooking. We both did our fair share of diaper changing, late night feedings and running kids to practices.

Now I'm not trying to say that our marriage is perfect. After 22 years, we've had our fair share of fights and arguments, and we've definitely faced many hard times, as most marriages do. When

Sean changed careers and became a mortgage broker, it really put a financial strain on our family. He was at a job that was 100% commission. The stress of closing a deal was massive in order for us to pay the bills. After all, I was just starting my massage career so I wasn't bringing in much money myself. We were living paycheck to paycheck. When we did argue, it was over finances. I am a natural worrier. It seems to come easy for me so being the one paying the bills, I saw our money dwindling fast and not enough coming in to replenish it. We both were feeling the stress and we knew that something had to give when we had to ask my dad to pay our mortgage one month. It wasn't what we wanted for our marriage or our family. A difficult conversation with one another and after a little luck, Sean changed careers again that would provide a more steady income. He did what he had to do and was always good at putting his family first like that.

At the time of his stroke, Sean was a Client Success Manager for an IT Medical Billing company based out of Tampa, Florida. Even though he had 15 years of experience in the field, he had only been with this company for 4 months. After working for the same company for over 12 years, we went through a very stressful time when his job was eliminated in June 2023. He was unemployed for 5 months, started with a new company and then lost that job 8 short months later. Stressful was an understatement of what he had been through and it was another time we experienced the dreaded financial strain. Although I do well financially as a Licensed Massage Therapist, Sean made significantly more than me. And he definitely felt that pressure. So, this opportunity with the Tampa Company had been a godsend and somewhere he was really excited about working, especially because he was also able to work for a former colleague.

Financial issues were just one thing we faced and conquered together as a couple. There's been addiction issues, loss of a parent, broken relationships with family members, and all the other things that make up the not-so-fun parts of a marriage. The real, raw and ugly side of a marriage. All the stuff that people don't post on social media. You know, the part of a marriage, where the sound of their breathing or how they chew their food drives you crazy! And the thoughts of suffocating them in their sleep when they're snoring is so loud and you are sleep deprived. If you've been married for any length of time, you know what I'm talking about. But the bottom line is yes, we've argued, but we've made up. We've disagreed, but we respect one another while doing so. We've made one another cry, but we apologize and comfort each other afterwards. We are raising 2, respectful young men and doing a damn good job of it if I say so myself. And that credit is being given to both of us. Our life, overall, has been wonderful. We have been a great team and we've survived a lot of shit together. And that's because we have leaned on one another as partners and as best friends and we've held true to our vows that we recited to one another on that October day. But that line in the vows of "in sickness and in health." Well, that's a line you say when you're in your 20s or 30s. And you think, *yes, when my partner is old and gray and their teeth have fallen out, I'm going to hold their hand and be with them during their sickness.* But when that vow comes to fruition when that person is still young, it holds a whole other meaning.

We're supposed to only be half way through our lives with a plethora of exciting adventures in our future – dream trips, watching our kids get married, babysitting grandchildren, retiring. All the things that you've dreamed about since the moment you said "I Do." But one day just changed all of that in an instant. I'm now going to have to prove that I really meant those 5 small words in that line of our vows. Because my husband is a 44-year-old stroke survivor and I am his wife.

CHAPTER 4

HOMEGIRLS

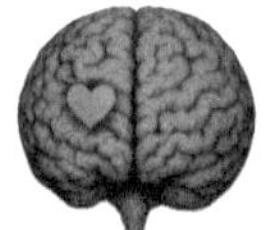

From a young age, I have been fortunate to have many girlfriends pass through my life. Some of those friends I lived next to as a child, but we lost contact once we moved away. Some would come in like a flash through the night and may only be a part of my life for a short time. Some were ladies that I grew attached to at work, even though our common bond was complaining about our jobs. Some girlfriends became my friends because our kids played ball together and we were together during the endless practices or weekend-long tournaments. And then there are those girlfriends that started out as family, but over time, became friends. It is so important to have all of these types of girlfriends. What's that saying?" People come into your life for a reason, a season or a lifetime." Relationships that we have with others can be temporary or long lasting, and they each serve a different purpose. I'd like to change just one word in that saying. "People come into your life for a reason, a season AND a lifetime." And those people are my Homegirls.

Kasey lovingly gave our group the name Homegirls when she moved to Georgia after graduating college. It was a way to separate us from her college friends and her new friends in Atlanta. We all gravitated toward the name and it has stuck with us over the years. These six women have played such an intricate role in my life, and going through this extremely difficult transition with Sean's stroke was no exception. They were some of the first on the scene to show up not just for Sean, but mostly for me. They anticipated my needs and were there without me even having to ask. But they also know me well enough and knew I wouldn't ask.

I originally met Kasey because we were on the dance team together in High School. Although we hung out in separate groups outside of school, she was someone I gravitated towards. Kasey can make any intense situation light-hearted and provides a guaranteed laugh. You'd think the physical distance between us would have made us grow apart over the years, but Kasey has always made her homegirls a priority. She's always been so wonderful about that, even if some of us haven't always reciprocated. There's never been a lack of effort on her part to keep her relationships thriving and it is one of my favorite traits about her.

Sara and I met in middle school and she was one of the few kids that moved on to the same high school as me. Seeing a familiar face on the first day of 9th grade helped with the first day jitters. Even though we knew each other before, we didn't truly start becoming friends until then. Since we had a base to our relationship, the friendship grew fast. She became one of my closest friends early on. She is a bubbly personality in a tiny frame and she's a guaranteed good time whenever she comes around. She's feisty but kind and she's got one of those loud, contagious laughs that you simply can't help but gravitate towards.

Then came Jill. Jill and I first met in freshman Algebra. Our last names were right next to each other alphabetically, so all the classes we had together, we'd end up sitting next to one another. She was a little more daring, if you will, than I was. I tend to be more of a rule-follower and a goody two shoes. She was not and I liked that about her. Don't get me wrong, we both excelled in school and cared very much about doing a good job, but this is also the same girl that paid me to say my first curse word. It was that moment that began a life-long friendship. I don't want to say she was a bad influence on me, but she definitely pushed my boundaries in a good way and allowed me to transform into a new version of myself. If Jill is around, you're going to have fun and she refuses to accept otherwise.

Melissa and I met my sophomore year of high school, but she went to a different school than I did. She started attending the church that I was going to at the time, and from the moment we met, we just had an instant connection. We bonded over our love to dance and our love for the Herndon brothers. So much so, we were determined that our friendship would eventually make us sister-in-laws! We were foolish young girls to say the least. So like most high school relationships, our love for the brothers faded, but our love towards one another only grew stronger. I brought her into my group of friends, and thankfully, she's never left.

Amanda and I also met in high school. We were honestly never really that close during that time as we hung out in separate groups. Amanda and Kasey had always been very close though and we all just kind of morphed into one group towards the end of our senior year. Looking back, I actually can't believe it took as long as it did because now I can't imagine Amanda not being there. She's got a hard exterior that can sometimes come off scary and you know exactly what she's thinking because it's impossible to hide all the expressions on her face. But she will fight ruthlessly for the people she loves and she's not afraid to stand up to anyone on their behalf. She is a friend that you want to have in your corner and I'm lucky I have her in mine.

Kelly joined our group last. Although she went to high school with all of us, she was a year younger and had her own group of friends during that time. She's always known everyone though so it wasn't a hard transition when she joined the group later on. Kelly is blunt and honest and doesn't sugar coat things, but her heart is big. She'd drop everything to help without the slightest hesitation. Oh, and did I mention that she also happens to be my cousin? So as far as she and I are concerned, there has never been a time she wasn't my best friend.

The bond that I share with these women is unbreakable. You can only imagine what we've been through together after three decades of friendship. High school break-ups, followed up by stalking our exes and their new girlfriends. That was Sara's specialty. She was a pro at that before there were cell phones and social media. If you needed to hack an email password or dress in black and spy on your ex from afar, she was your girl.

Then there were the college years. While Jill and Sara went to University of Louisville, the rest of us went to Western Kentucky University. Although Kasey was the only one who survived all four years there we managed to make the most of it during the short time we were all together. Fraternity parties, late nights in the dorm room, and make-out sessions with strangers. We did it all and did it together. There were more boyfriends that came and went and someone was always there to help mend the broken hearts. That was the good part about there being seven of us. We may not have always been there at the same time, but you could always count on at least one girl to show up when you needed them.

Our early 20s were greeted with weddings, babies and new homes. We all had a closet full of bridesmaids dresses and bachelorette party outfits since for a while, it seemed like that's all we were doing. The bridal showers soon turned into baby showers and we were welcoming little ones into our family. Our group of friends continued to grow as our husbands and later, our children, became friends. There were big moves and sometimes, even bigger job promotions. Some of us branched out and owned our own businesses while others went back to school to take different career paths. We celebrated one another's accomplishments and were each other's biggest cheerleaders. There wasn't a single big moment in all of our lives that we missed.

Unfortunately, with the celebrations of life, there were also heartbreak and tears that would intertwine with the good times. The difficult times are the true testament of our friendship. Several of us went through a time of losing a parent. Myself, Amanda and Melissa have all lost our dads, while Jill and Kasey have lost their moms. It's inevitable that those days will come, but it is always a little more comforting when you have your people by your side to help you get through it. There have been parenting challenges, divorces, family drama, and even disagreements amongst our own group. We learned to grow with one another, accept the changes and lean on each other to get us through the bumps, and sometimes mountains of life.

We've done countless girls trips and traveled all over the country and beyond. Those trips are necessary to get through life. They allowed us to have a break from our spouses, children, and jobs. The most difficult decision on those trips is deciding what kind of wine to have with dinner. We spend that time laughing and crying and bringing up old memories and stories. We share our worries and give advice. We argue over who is the funny one and who posts the most on social media. Our cheeks and abs hurt from the laughter that helps burn the calories from all the food and drinks we consume. It makes for a wonderful reset and they never last long enough.

Ironically, in all the years of doing these trips, we've never been able to have all seven of us go. Inevitably, someone has an obstacle that keeps them from attending. But this year, we were going to all be making the trip. I was actually in the process of narrowing down the lodging and flights for a girls trip to Montana in September 2025, in celebration of the year we all turn 45 years old. But that planning came to a screeching halt on that January day.

Kelly got the call from Ricky about Sean, and she took on the difficult role of informing the rest of the group. The year of an epic trip was quickly replaced by just being there for a friend in desperate need of her homegirls. And that friend was me.

A few months after Sean's stroke, Melissa sent us a social media reel in our group chat. I swear I've watched it no less than 10 times. It was a woman talking on a podcast about an older lady that read this poem at a recent bridal shower that she attended. Anticipating that the poem would be about marriage, it wasn't. Instead, it was a poem titled "Keep Your Girlfriends," author unknown.

Keep Your Girlfriends

I sat on a porch in Waycross, Georgia on a summer day drinking ice tea and visiting with my mother. "Don't forget your girlfriends," my mother advised, clinking the ice cubes in her glass. No matter how much you love your husband, you are still going to need girlfriends. Remember to go places with them now and then and do things with them. Remember that girlfriends are not only friends, but sisters, daughters and other relatives too. "What a funny piece of advice," I thought. Hadn't I just gotten married? Hadn't I just joined the couple world? I was now a married woman, for goodness sake, not a young girl who needed girlfriends." But I listened to my mom. I kept contact with my girlfriends and made more each year. As the years tumbled by one after another, gradually I came to understand that my mom really knew what she was talking about. Here is what I know about girlfriends. Girlfriends bring casseroles and scrub your bathroom when you need help. Girlfriends keep your children and keep your secrets. Girlfriends give advice when you ask for it, sometimes you take it, sometimes you don't. Girlfriends don't always tell you that you're right but they are usually honest. Girlfriends still love you even though they don't agree with your choices. Girlfriends laugh with you and don't need canned jokes to start the laughter. Girlfriends pull you out of your jams. Girlfriends will give a party for your son or daughter when they get married or have a baby, in whichever order that comes. Girl-

friends are there for you in an instant when the hard times come. Girl-friends listen to you when you lose a job or a friend. Girlfriends listen when your children break your heart. Girlfriends listen when your parents' minds and bodies fail. Girlfriends cry with you when someone that you love dies. My daughters, sisters, family and friends bless my life. When we began this adventure we had no idea of the incredible joys or sorrows that lay ahead. Nor did we know how much we need each other. So, keep your girlfriends.

These words ring so true with my relationships with not just my Homegirls, but the other powerful women that have come into my life for "a season, a reason or a lifetime." I truly had no idea how much I would need them all, especially during this time accepting this new version of life with Sean. My sister, Kimberly, who has been my constant from the moment she was born. Ali, the person responsible for the life that I have with Sean and my boys. My friend and boss, Laura. Not only has she been an amazing boss, especially during this time caring for Sean, but a friend I can depend on for sound advice and a laugh. There have been count-less others and I am thankful for each and every one of them. They have all played a part in shaping me into the person I am today and I just hope that I've made a fraction of that same impact on them. My advice is the same as the old lady in the poem, keep your girlfriends. But I'll add one more statement to that. Get your-self at least one Homegirl.

CHAPTER 5
BETWEEN BEEPS AND PRAYERS

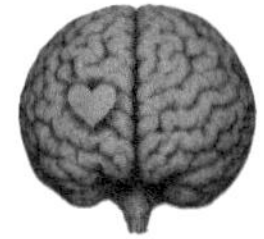

We had about a twenty minute drive to U of L Hospital. Ricky, Sean's best friend, drove my car while I sat in the passenger seat and Austin in the back. I thought of Chris. I thought of my Dad. I thought of Landon. And I prayed for Sean. Harder than I've ever prayed before. I just couldn't lose him. Ricky and I came up with a plan to get the word out to our closest family and friends.

"Call Mike and Karen back. Call Sean's brother, Joey, and call Kelly." I muttered to Ricky.

I knew Kelly would be a good center contact for all my important groups of people. She could obviously get the word out to all the family, but being a part of the Homegirls group, she could let them know too. She also knew my boss, Laura. And I knew she would take care of letting them all know without even being instructed to do so. Kelly and I have very similar personalities, so I had no doubt she'd take care of things.

Unbeknownst to me, Ricky had already arranged for his son, Michael, to get on the road to go pick up Landon in Tennessee. And I had to be the one to make that call to tell him. I wasn't going to put that off on anyone else. I picked up my phone and texted Landon.

> Can you get away somewhere quiet and call me?
> It's urgent.

To my surprise, it only took him a minute to respond. With shaky hands and voice, I dialed his number.

I knew as soon as I heard his voice, I'd probably break down. Sure enough, I did. "Landon, dad has had a stroke." I barely got the words out but he was able to decipher them. His voice turned from light heartedness to the same panic that mine was in just an hour before.

"What?! Are you kidding me?" I heard his tears through my own. "I'm leaving now. I'm on my way home." Within five seconds he had already decided on a plan. I knew that was exactly how he was going to react. He is your eldest child's personality, through and through. I always say, he's the boy version of me, so I wasn't surprised at his reaction to this news. It would have been exactly how I would have reacted.

I managed to talk over him and interrupt his plans before he could hang up on me and get on the road. "Michael is already on his way to get you. You don't need to be driving. He'll bring you straight to the hospital." Not only was Michael Landon's cousin, but his best friend. Michael had been through a lot of difficult times in his life and Landon had always been there for him. Now it was time for Michael to be there for Landon. That eased my heart somewhat that he'd have someone to be with during the drive.

We pulled into the hospital parking garage and attempted to navigate ourselves through the hospital to find the ER. My heart was racing. Still every thought possible running through my head. Ricky stayed outside to start the calls to everyone. Austin and I got into the ER waiting room. Once again, we beat the ambulance there. We stood to the side as there wasn't an empty chair in the room. Being in the downtown location and not in the best area of the city, that ER has a little bit of everything. I actually welcomed the distraction of people watching while I waited. Lines of patients and their families entering the ER through metal detectors. It probably isn't uncommon for someone to sneak in a knife or gun. There were guys in bar fights, being escorted by their girlfriends, with blood dripping out of their noses and eyes all bruised up. Kids with snotty noses, homeless people with hacking coughs and addicts pacing around having conversations with themselves.

Everyone was looking to get immediate help. The damp air and smell of sickly patients filled the air. It wasn't long before the security guard approached me, notifying me that Sean had arrived. They escorted us back, down a hall into a smaller waiting room with not quite so many distractions as the main one. Slowly, people started arriving. First, it was Joey and his family, Ricky's wife, then Mike and Karen. They all entered the room with solemn faces and worry in their voices. Each embrace started a new trail of tears. We were all scared and had no idea what was to come. Melissa and Amanda showed up shortly afterwards, confirming that Kelly did exactly what I knew she would do. I remember being shocked to see them there when I entered back into the room from calling Sean's boss. I had only been there myself for maybe 30 minutes.

Honestly my first instinct was to say "What are you doing here? You don't need to be here now. I'm fine." After all, I was very overwhelmed in that moment and was simply trying to gather my thoughts on what was even occurring. I didn't really want to talk to anyone. But that's the perk of being friends for so long. They already knew that. They simply hugged me tightly, gave me comforting smiles, and sat quietly in the waiting room chairs. I simply just needed their presence, and they were giving that to me without me even knowing that was what I needed.

The Neuro doctor on duty popped in and asked to speak with me privately. My heart sank once again. *What now? And why privately? This couldn't be good.* But we weren't exactly in a positive situation here.

The doctor started in, "I've ordered an MRI for Sean so we can get a closer look at what is going on. We've also ordered an angiogram to be done first thing next week. That is a type of x-ray that allows us to see his blood vessels more in detail that we cannot see in the other medical imaging scans. His blood pressure is dangerously high so we are monitoring that closely by putting in an A-line. This will give us his blood pressure as it is in the moment. We are going to transfer him to the ICU and you can expect for him to be here at least a week. As of right now, we don't think surgery will be required and we want to avoid that at all costs. The brain bleed is deep on the left side and we would have to go through healthy brain tissue to extract it, which could potentially cause more problems. As long as things don't worsen, over time the body and brain will naturally absorb the excess blood. But we will have to closely monitor him to make sure the pressure in the brain isn't getting worse because of the bleed. The next several days will be the most crucial for the swelling and bleeding."

The thought of Chris interrupted my thoughts with the doctor's words. *His brain swelling. His coma. His fate. In this hospital. On their ICU floor.* I just couldn't comprehend that I had to go through all that again. I just COULDN'T lose Sean. I refused.

"Ma'am?" She must have been able to tell that I started to zone out. "Ma'am, did Sean do any hard drugs?" *What?! How could she ask me that?* I mean, he enjoyed the daily beer or bourbon and had been a nicotine user since high school, but hard drugs? No. Sean didn't do that and never had. She confirmed that there weren't any signs in his blood work showing that he did, but it was very concerning to have someone as young as Sean to have a stroke this severe.

"Usually, patients that have a hemorrhagic stroke at his age will be because they use cocaine or similar drugs. It is less than a 5% chance for someone his age to experience this." I stood there dumbfounded. *So, if Sean didn't do drugs, how was he "picked" to be the less than the 5%?* The stinging in my eyes started back up. This wasn't fair. This had to be a nightmare.

The doctor gave me a comforting shoulder tap and finished with, "We're going to take good care of him. Would you like to come see him before we transfer him to the ICU?" I nodded, headed back to the small waiting room and gave everyone an update. They allowed all of us to go see him.

Austin decided he wanted to go this time. We all walked in line formation in silence through the crowded hallway back to Sean's small room. We dodged patients laying on gurneys in the hall and medical equipment around every corner. The hustle and bustle of the nurses and doctors scurrying through the halls of the busy ER. We turned around the corner and entered Sean's room. I rushed to his side and grabbed his now swollen hand. Karen went to his other side. I knew how I felt as his wife, but the thought of looking at my baby boy lying in the bed unconscious was unimaginable. My heart broke for her in that moment. I looked up, and the Troklus men were staring at Sean wiping tears from their eyes. Austin only peered in the doorway and observed from afar. I worried for him too.

The doctor pulled up an image of Sean's CT. Although we weren't medical staff, it was clear to see in the images that Sean's bleed was bad. It had caused the left side to swell over the mid-line of the brain and into the right side. At that time, I didn't know exactly what it meant, but I knew it probably wasn't good. We all said our messages to Sean, some whispering in his ear and others silently to themselves. I closed my eyes tightly, tears squeezing out of my eyes and down my cheeks. I prayed to God again to bring him back to me.

We were up in his ICU room by 10 that evening. Everyone went home for the night but I stayed by his side. No way I could leave, nor did I want to. I sat there in the hard lounge chair that I was told was an actual upgrade to what they had just a few months prior. The room was small, with barely enough room for the bed, my lounger and all the medical equipment. The beeping noises and alarms attached to the machines were sounding the entire time. I sat staring at the monitor on the wall that tracked his oxygen, blood pressure and heart rate. I couldn't pull my eyes away from it.

A nurse walked in to check on him and said to me, "You'll drive yourself crazy watching those monitors. You're going to have to look away or get out of the room at some point." I forced a grin. I knew she was just trying to be helpful. Sean laid still in the bed while the ventilator breathed for him and a trach feeding tube gave him his required nutrients. I held his hand and didn't let go. My adrenaline was coming down and my eyes were still burning, not just from the tears but from the exhaustion of the evening. It was all catching up with me. Landon was still a few hours away and I wanted to be up when he arrived. I just needed to hug him, for him and for me.

The nurses on the ICU are each assigned only two patients since everyone there has to be monitored so closely, so there was someone coming in every thirty minutes. They started conducting stimulus tests during those check-ins. They would lower the sedation drip, yell his name and pinch and twist all over his body to try and get a response. It seemed like the entire unit could hear the yelling. Everyone could hear her. Well, everyone except Sean. He would give no response.

Landon and Michael arrived around 3:30 a.m. I actually managed to doze off in the hard chair, when I was awakened by Landon tapping me on the shoulder. "Hey Mom." It was the voice I needed to hear. I was so glad he was there. He, too, looked exhausted. The worry and even a little guilt on his face that he couldn't be there sooner.

The nurse came back in the room for another stimulus check. "Does he have a nickname by chance?" she asked.

"Trok," I answered. He got the nickname during his high school years playing baseball, when they shortened the last name Troklus. The nickname Trok was almost a right of passage with the men of the family. Mike had the same nickname growing up, then Joey. Sean was next in line and sure enough, Landon's friends started calling him Trok as well. But Sean's closest friends still call him Trok to this day.

I stood next to him with Landon on the other side, while the nurse started her pinching routine and yelled "TROK!" And just like that, his eyes opened up slowly and shut right back. Landon swore he looked right at him. *Were my prayers already starting to be answered?* I didn't know but I was living on hope at that moment, so that's what I chose to believe. Landon went home and I got myself as comfortable as possible in what looked to be my bed for the unknown future. As I drifted back off to sleep to the beeps of the machines, I said one more prayer for good measure. Tomorrow was a new day, which I welcomed because today had been a nightmare.

––––––

The word about Sean's stroke spread like wildfire and by the time I woke up on the first morning at U of L Hospital, my phone was blowing up with texts, emails and Facebook messages. That over-whelming feeling crept back in with a vengeance and the thought of responding to everyone was just too much to handle. I knew they were just concerned and worried, but I just didn't have the mental strength to respond to each of them.

Ricky arrived back at the hospital early that morning, greeting me with a much-needed cup of coffee. The two hours of broken sleep I got throughout the night wasn't going to be enough to get me through the day that was ahead of me. I was reluctant to take Sean's status to social media, but after talking with Ricky, agreed that it was the easiest and quickest way to get his status out to everyone. Not to mention, it wouldn't hurt to have more prayer warriors on our side. I felt like God was already tired of hearing just my voice.

The first full day at U of L was full of poking and prodding and tests. The medical team were still trying to figure out what caused the stroke. In addition to multiple doctors and nurses, there were now respiratory therapists added to the mix. They would come in to check his ventilator and brush his teeth. There was an echocardiogram to check the strength of his heart, an MRI to get a more detailed image of the brain damage, new medication drips, changing out the trach tube to a feeding tube up the nose, check, check, check.

It was a constant revolving door of harassment. The results from the echo showed thickening of the heart tissue which told the physicians that he probably had undiagnosed hypertension, also known as high blood pressure, for a while now. As they monitored all of his IVs, they had to remove his wedding band. The fluids were filling his body causing him to swell and he could no longer keep it on his finger. I took his ring and put it on my necklace to keep it close.

Stimulus checks continued to be done every hour. It was the same drill – sedative IVs turned down, yelling, pinching and squeezing. Sean's eyes would force open but would then quickly close. It looked like the strength it took to just open his eyes was nearly an impossible feat. He started responding to local stimuli. I guess the forceful pinching was starting to piss him off. He would move his left hand towards the area being tortured. He started responding to small commands, wiggling toes and tiny hand squeezes on the left side only and gave a small, half way thumbs up.

By the end of the day, Austin came to visit during one of the checks. The nurse came in but decided to turn up the intensity of the pinching and gave it an extra twist. Sean's eyes shot open and we thought he was going to hit her. It was a bit humorous but also exciting to see some aggression behind his responses. That being said, the right side of his body remained completely still.

CHAPTER 6
GO CARDS!

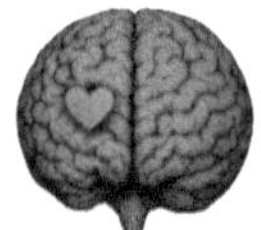

here was a constant flow of visitors coming up to visit Sean. Although there was supposed to be a maximum of two guests in the room at a time, there would always be a few more to sneak back. When I wasn't in the room with Sean, I'd venture out into the ICU waiting room. It was a bit of a change of scenery, but my mental status didn't take much of a break. Everyone that came to visit wanted to hear the story of how it happened, what could have caused it, and how things are going. I had to relive that day over and over as I repeated the story to each visitor. With every telling of the story, I'd start crying again, each time draining my energy just a little more. I found it comforting, though, that whenever I'd start crying, Landon would just appear. He was constantly checking on me. He was being and doing what Sean would usually do for me. Landon was stepping up and filling in the man of the house role. It wasn't any surprise to me that he was reacting that way, but it also made me worry about how he was going to be once it was time to return to college. He was already missing the second week of the semester.

Landon tried talking me into going home for the night since it had been three days since I left the hospital. At that point, the smells and germs of the hospital felt like they were deep into my pores. My scalp was itchy and my skin was dry. I was so tired, I'd have periods of delirium. My stomach was growling and having a full-on irritated conversation with me about not giving it anything to eat. But in the midst of everything going on with Sean, I just kept forgetting. And really, I didn't want to. I was getting grief about not eating from all my girlfriends who were watching my food intake closely which was never satisfactory to their standards. At one point while I was in the ICU waiting room, Jill even took a picture of me taking a bite to send it to the girls' group texts. I know they were worried about me, but I was worried about Sean and Sean only. Taking care of myself just wasn't a priority because that meant I had to leave Sean's side and it just wasn't worth it. But the thought of a shower and a bed did sound appealing. So I agreed with Landon to go home. Plus, I knew he probably wanted to have some time alone with his dad.

I rode with Mike and Karen on the way back home. Their temporary bedroom that was in our basement for when they would visit had now become a permanent bedroom for the unforeseen future. More of their clothes and belongings had moved in for good. It was added stress of having additional people in the house, but I knew I needed them. And luckily, I do get along with my in-laws so that is a silver lining of the living situation. I sluggishly walked into the bedroom and noticed there were still stickers on the floor from the back of the pads that were put on Sean's chest by the EMS crew. Flashbacks of everything came flooding back. I wanted to go back to the hospital with Sean. I didn't want to be there.

What if something happened overnight while I was gone? What if he woke up and I wasn't there?

I tried not to let my thoughts take over. I got in the shower and as the hot water fell on my skin, the intensity of the last days and hours caught up with me and the breakdown happened. I let it all out. I felt safe to do so because no one was around to feel sorry for me or worry about me or judge me. I didn't have to be concerned about staying strong or hiding my tears. I was alone and I took full advantage of the situation. It was a nice relief to just let all the emotions fall out. I pulled myself together and headed to bed. But the comfortable bed I was crawling into almost felt colder than the ICU room. I looked at the empty pillow lying to the right of me. Instead of Sean, it was a box of Kleenex and a stack of cards that people gave me when visiting. I had several nights sleeping alone in our bed over the years when Sean would travel for work, but this was totally different. I felt alone and scared. I couldn't help but wonder if and when Sean would one day replace the box of Kleenex. I opened up my phone and took the time to read each of the texts and comments that had been sent to me, since I couldn't focus enough to read while at the hospital. I wrote a "Sean Status" update on Facebook, cried a little more and fell fast asleep while tightly holding on to his wedding band that was around my neck.

Ricky and I arrived back at the hospital first thing the next morning. I had my coffee in one hand and my overnight bag in the other. Landon and I decided we would alternate nights staying all night with Sean and tonight would be my turn. We all agreed that we never wanted to leave him alone. Landon awoke when we arrived and was still groggy from sleeping in the hard lounger.

They started the process of weaning Sean off the stronger drugs and replacing them with a less sedative medication that put him more in a deep sleep versus a coma-like state. The ventilator was still in, but they were hopeful it could come out soon, as long as they could see further progress of him staying awake more on his own without stimulation. The respiratory therapist said he was taking a few deep breaths and gave a cough which is a good sign. By late morning they tried turning all the sedatives off to see how he'd do on his own.

Luckily, Sean's amazing ICU physician, who was also a Neurosurgeon and the Director of Neurotrauma, was aggressive with her care. She was like the queen of the department and seemed to not only have the respect from her patients, but also her staff. Dr. Queen was an intelligent and confident bad ass and I couldn't have loved her more. When she spoke, we'd all just hang on every word because she would speak with so much self-assurance. She was assertive, but humble at the same time. So even though he wasn't staying awake quite as long as they hoped, she was ready to push him along and take the vent out! I was a little shocked by the decision but also had faith in Dr. Queen and her decisions when it came to Sean's care. And the relief of seeing one less thing connected to his body was comforting. They immediately tried doing another stimulus check on him and he wasn't following any of the commands. He'd get angry, but wouldn't try hitting them away so that is an issue they wanted to see improve.

Now that the vent was out, it was time to bring in yet another therapist. Timing is crucial in situations like this one, and I was told time and time again that the fact that I arrived home when I did may have saved Sean's life. The second timing miracle was with Homegirl Sara. Sara just so happened to be the lead Speech Therapist at U of L Hospital. She made the schedules for her whole staff and herself and she mostly worked in the ICU unit with the stroke patients, so it was a clear move to assign herself to Sean. She had been looking to make a career move within the organization for some time now, but something continued to keep her from doing so. It was all about the timing and it was Sean that kept her in that position. She obviously had no idea that is why she stayed, but God knew. I truly believe that she was meant to stay on that ICU unit just to help care for Sean and comfort me.

Seeing someone you adore and love like a sister care for the most important person in your life was such an honor to witness and I was so extremely thankful that God's timing allowed Sara to do just that. She was not only a comfort blanket for me, but she was a familiar face for Sean as he started opening his eyes. She bounced into his room. She was "friend Sara" when she walked in greeting me with a hug and breakfast. She was one of the girls on a mission to see me eat anything. Then she quickly turned into "Speech Sara," going over to Sean and doing her evaluation. She explained that now that the vent was out, they are going to start analyzing his swallowing before he can start orally eating or drinking anything. She will slowly start introducing him to ice chips and then move on from there and eventually perform a swallow test on him. But there were still several things Sean would have to do before we got to that point.

Sara was able to get the swallow tests scheduled within a few days and he passed "with restrictions." That meant he would graduate to a liquid only diet for the time being but had to keep the feeding tube in to help supplement the remaining calories. The goal was to get him to 2000 calories per day. So Ensure protein shakes, sherbet, pudding and chicken broth would be on the menu for the next several meals. By the next day, he was doing well enough to get the feeding tube out and was on the road to graduating to more solid foods. He was slowly starting to look like himself again as another tube would be taken out of his body.

There continued to be a few exciting moments throughout the day as he started opening his eyes more. He seemed to keep them open a little longer when someone he knew came to visit and would talk to him. Dr. Queen came in with another update. The MRI results came back showing no new changes. But we aren't in the clear. The next three days are still very critical as that is the biggest chance for additional swelling of the brain. An angiogram was scheduled for the following day to rule out any other possible underlying issues. His blood pressure was still very high, and they were having a hard time keeping it down. He was maxed out on IV blood pressure medication so they had to add on another one. She warned me that this time in the ICU and the early stages of recovery would be a lot of "one step forward, two steps back" and "one day at a time" and "It's not a sprint, it's a marathon." If I heard it once, I heard it a million times. They probably wanted to make sure that it was soaking in and I wasn't creating false hope. But it was hard not to want Sean to be the exception to the rule. Maybe he'd be the miracle patient that came in from a severe stroke but two days later would just wake up, stand up and walk right out of here. So to avoid that, Dr. Queen and her team made sure to constantly keep us up to date, explaining things in great detail and staying in the room until every question was answered. If I started getting a glazed look on my face, she simply took my phone out of my hand and typed the notes in for me. She was extremely comforting but kept things realistic for me and the family. As scared as we all were, we also knew he was in good hands.

These doctors and nurses were the best of the best in my opinion. Sean and I had always been U of L Cardinal fans when it came to sports, especially when going against our rivals at University of Kentucky. But the phrase "Go Cards!" took on a whole new meaning within 48 hours of being at that hospital. I was now cheering on the U of L neurosurgeons, ICU physicians, nurses and therapists. The sports teams didn't even hold a candle to them because they were the ones that I was putting my faith in to bring Sean back to me.

Around nightfall when visitors were leaving, the chatter out in the halls settled down and it was just him and I in the room again. Sean's blood sugar started dropping so they had to give him glucose. The sedative started wearing down causing him to become very restless and defiant. He was moving all around in the bed and began reaching with his left hand towards his face, pulling out the oxygen tube and yanking off the oxygen mask and then pulling out his feeding tube. That's when we were introduced to "the mitt." A large mitt that resembled a boxing glove was put on his left hand and would velcro around his wrist. The intention of this was to keep him from pulling things out, but because he was becoming a little more awake, he did not like the lack of movement that the mitt provided. He tried reaching for my hand and when he couldn't grab it, he aggressively wiped the mitt across his chest until he was able to maneuver it off. I wanted nothing more than to hold his hand as well. Precedex, a stronger sedative and analgesic, had to be given to him to try and calm him down. The more agitated he got, the higher his blood pressure would increase and would in turn also raise his heart rate. As I stood beside the bed, watching him fight what was going on with his body, I tried calming him down, but it only seemed to make things worse. He was confused and scared, and you could see it in his eyes.

The night nurse came in and sternly instructed me to not touch or talk to him. Seeing me and hearing my voice was only stimulating him, causing his stats to increase high enough that they couldn't get it under control. The mitt was put back on him, even tighter this time with restraints around his hand to hold it down to the bed. I wanted to be there for him more than anything. I not only wanted to hold his hand, but I wanted to crawl in the bed with him and wrap my body around his. Instead, the lights were all turned off and I had to sit quietly in the corner of the room, completely out of his sight. I sat there continuing to watch him struggle and silently started crying. He continued to move all around and managed to look through an opening in the top of the bed where he made eye contact with me. The begging for help in his eyes was unbearable to watch. He was trying to talk, but still nothing would come out except an occasional grunt. He didn't understand what was going on with him. I squeezed my eyes shut and silently said a prayer for calmness and stillness to just take over his body. Because we were both being tortured in the current state.

It took a little over an hour for the sedative to kick in, and possibly my prayer, and he finally started to doze off. His oxygen levels started dropping so they had to put him on a high-flow, which is a machine that helps to get more air to the lungs. His breathing was becoming more shallow and they needed to get his lungs to expand more. Although they told me there's no reason for great concern, their urgency at taking care of the matter told me otherwise.

My night was restless. I woke up often, checking on his vitals each time. By that point, I knew exactly where everything needed to be and what to look for. They kept the mitt on him all night but were able to release the arm restraint. The respiratory therapist was back bright and early to check his breathing. He said his chest sounded clear and oxygen levels were staying at 94. He'll slowly start weaning him off the high-flow when they feel his lungs can handle it. They also started turning the bed on, where it would shake vigorously for about twenty minutes. It is supposed to help loosen things up in his chest and keep things moving instead of settling in. That has started becoming as regular as the torturous stimulus checks. The angiogram was scheduled for later that day so they changed out his oxygen from the high-flow since that machine cannot go back to the room where the procedure will take place.

Dr. Queen came back later that day to check on him and gave us the results from the angiogram. It was a sigh of relief when she reported that the test came back showing no further damage or additional issues of any kind. She confirmed that the stroke was caused from undiagnosed hypertension. In true Dr. Queen fashion, although she was happy with the results from the angiogram, she is still preparing us that there are some difficult days ahead as they try to take him off oxygen and sedatives. Doing this all while keeping his blood pressure in check was going to be a challenge. She said during this time, and especially in younger men, there can be a lot of agitation and combativeness. This transition can not only be difficult for Sean, but even more so for the family as it is a side of Sean that is unlike him but very well may rear its ugly head.

"I can now confirm that the stroke was caused from undiagnosed hypertension" she said with her typical confidence, and it was the one line that stood out to me. That one statement rang in my ears.

As relieved as I was to get the news that there weren't any other underlying issues, I was mad. It was the first time that that emotion pushed its way through. I had been getting on Sean for the last few years about taking care of himself and that meant going to get regular check-ups at the doctor. I tried to lead by example by getting all of my check-ups. Not just lab work with my primary care physician, but visits to the gynecologist, mammogram, dentist and dermatologist for a full body check. I didn't enjoy it by any means, but I knew the importance. But that didn't seem to persuade him to make any appointments. After all, he was young and active so what was so urgent to get checked?! After two years of nicely asking, I ended up just playing the part of a nagging wife who bugged him about it and that wasn't enjoyable for either of us and definitely wasn't getting us anywhere. He was irritated with me because I wouldn't let it go and I was annoyed that he wouldn't just go. It was a constant cycle. About a year ago, he started complaining of frequent headaches. Then it got to the point where the only medication that would touch it was Excedrin Migraine. They would come on a couple times a week and all he'd do was whine about them.

I would sarcastically respond with, "hey, here's a thought…instead of just bitching, why don't you go to the doctor?" He'd quickly shrug it off and chalk it up to allergies and sinuses. After all, we do live in an allergy prone state. But being fed up again, I tried one last tactic. Guilt. It was less than 24 hours before Sean's stroke. We were home alone and I calmly went to him and said, "I'm going to bring something up and I don't want you to get defensive."

"Yes?" with a very questionable expression. I'm sure he really didn't want to hear what I had to say.

"I have been very patient with you over the last couple of years in asking you to go to the doctor. I lost my dad at a young age and I can't help but think I could have had him around longer had he not been so stubborn and gone for regular doctor check-ups. I want you around until we are old and gray. Please just go to the doctor this year?" I guess that finally got through to him.

Hesitantly but in an affirming tone, he replied with "yes, I will make an appointment to go to the doctor." That was his response the night before we ended up in this hospital. So, yeah, I was mad. I was mad at him for not going sooner then maybe his blood pressure would have been "diagnosed" instead of "undiagnosed." I was mad at myself for not thinking of the guilt trip tactic long before. The what-if scenarios were playing out over and over. But one thing I knew for sure was his days of not going to doctors were a thing of the past and he was going to be making up for lost time now. He had many appointments in his future.

———

It was day five of being in the ICU. I was learning very quickly that all of this is a roller coaster. One minute we're up and celebrating a milestone and the next we're crashing down from a new scare that popped up. Sean's neurosurgeon that performed the angiogram greeted Karen and I when we arrived that morning. He was a young-looking doctor, maybe in his mid 30s. Almost too young to be a neurosurgeon. His dark complexion and tall, thin build stood in the doorway of Sean's room. Just like Dr. Queen, he reeked of confidence, but his confidence was paired with a touch of cologne and a bright smile. I couldn't pronounce his last name, but I heard Isaac so I humorously referred to him from that moment on as "Hot Isaac." I amused myself with the nickname and I was open to any little bit of comedic relief I could find during all this.

Hot Isaac told us that he was happy with the progress Sean was making, but getting the blood pressure and oxygen levels under control continued to be a challenge. They set specific parameters that he must meet before moving to the next step. Blood pressure must stay at 150 or below, he was to increase oxygen levels on his own and get off all drips before moving out of the ICU. And at that point and time, they didn't know how long that would take. It was a balancing act of decreasing the blood pressure, moving to oral medications through the feeding tube and increasing oxygen levels. They are currently set on higher settings from the high-flow machine so they have to wean him off of that too. They lowered the sedative medication as well, which is causing him to be more alert overall. He started moving but everything is in slow motion. He would reach up to rub his hair and scratch his head. Then he'd start reaching for my hand, and giving it a slight squeeze with his left hand. It was a weak squeeze but a squeeze nonetheless and although he still wasn't talking, I knew he could hear us and hear me. Every now and then, his eyes would slightly open up and then quickly shut. It was small steps, but they were encouraging steps.

Throughout the early afternoon, his oxygen levels continued to drop despite bringing down all the volume levels of fluids he was being administered. The respiratory therapist changed him over to a bi-pap machine to help push the fluids out of his lungs. If his oxygen didn't start to improve quickly, they were going to have to trach him again. He couldn't remain at 87 for long. Things started to turn around and within an hour, his blood oxygen level started to go back up. They continued to lower the blood pressure drip medications while switching over to the feeding tube from IV medications.

It was around 10 o'clock that evening the day ended on a high note. Now that the sedatives were completely turned off, he was able to finally give the doctor a hand squeeze, thumbs up and a high five on command. After the scares from the day with the oxygen and blood pressure, this was like witnessing a miracle. There started the stinging in my eyes again that was becoming a very familiar feeling.

"Keep going babe. You're doing awesome! Don't give up." I said to him with an encouraging smile.

With that, he slowly moved his left arm and put his hand up on my shoulder. I tried not to squeal with excitement. He then, with purpose, moved his hand down my arm and to my back, pulling me in towards him. I met him the rest of the way, wrapping my arms around him and breaking down once again. His arm loosely laid on my back as he still could not hold me like I craved to be held. But it was that purposeful hug that was going to get me up to tackle yet another day.

That one hug was so powerful to not just me, but to Sean too. As he approached the end of the critical stage and was becoming a little more aware, we started to see pretty good improvement. He was recognizing more faces, reaching out to give a fist bump or high five, waving good-bye and was giving facial expressions of his own. They started doing short fifteen minute physical therapy sessions to simply try and get him to keep his balance long enough to sit up on his own. But those short sessions would wear him out and he'd sleep for several hours afterwards. Sara continued to see him both when scheduled and when she'd just pop in to visit me. A few ice chips were turning into trying to brush his teeth and still continuing to try and make a noise of any kind. But still nothing was coming out. He also started to realize that he couldn't move anything on the right side of his body. I know he had to be confused but couldn't even ask the questions.

There would be times I would just sit in his room and just stare. Sometimes it would be at him, a lot of times it would be at the monitors and occasionally somewhere off into space. I felt so help-less. I decided to ask his doctors if I could give him a massage. At least let me use my expertise to possibly help him and keep my mind busy as well. I got the approval from them, so I started giving him daily lymphatic drainage massages. Although I didn't have a lot of experience giving these types of massages, I still had some knowledge and knew it would be beneficial in Sean's case. With him continuing to be so swollen from all the fluids, this massage technique is designed to help the natural movement of lymph fluid through the body and can help eliminate toxins and excess fluids from the tissues. I also incorporated some stretching in his limbs and range of motion in the joints, especially on his right side since it wasn't getting any movement. Sean always begged to get massages from me and now I was begging to give him one. Although I didn't get a verbal thank you, I was getting small hand squeezes instead.

They really worked on getting his circadian rhythm fixed. A lot of people that come in from stroke get their days and nights mixed up so it was crucial to talk in normal voices and keep the lights on during the day and quiet and dark at night. He started experiencing what they called "ICU Delirium" as well. This consists of confusion, disorientation and even hallucinations. It wouldn't be uncommon to look over and see him grabbing at the imaginary spots in the sky. Agitation was another side effect, which he shared a great deal of irritation towards The Mitt! They'd put it on and he'd try and take it off as soon as they'd walk out of the room. It was a bit amusing because it was like watching a defiant child. The more they turned down the sedatives, the more restless he'd get overall.

———

After a little over a week in the ICU, Landon approached me and was ready to discuss what the near future would look like for him. I took my wife hat off and replaced it with my mom hat. I was ready to focus on Landon and his needs. I was immediately taken back to my time in college where I was faced with a similar decision when I got that call from my dad saying my mom had left. My instinct was to immediately come home, and I knew Landon was battling with the same instinct. I was prepared to not only come to him with mom advice, but also with the experience of being faced with the same decision when I was his age. Although I didn't regret my decision to return home to help my dad after the semester ended, I wanted something different for Landon.

He started, "I think I'm going to go back to school if that's okay with you?" I was pleasantly surprised. He was firm with his words, but also had an undertone of asking for my permission. I had already been given the heads up by a few friends that came to me saying that Landon was really struggling on what to do and was scared he'd make the wrong decision. He was being brought to tears with the difficulty of the decision lying ahead of him... continue to focus on his future or drop out and come home to help his family. But I knew exactly what I needed to say.

"Absolutely! I think that would be a great idea." He needed to hear that I was going to be okay with him returning to school, and I made sure to respond with enthusiasm. "Austin and I will be fine. I promise to keep you updated every day with what is going on with dad. I won't keep you in the dark." I continued. "I'm really proud of you for making this tough decision. I think it's very important for you to try and stay focused at school."

"I still plan to come home and help with dad on the weekends or whenever you need me." He was talking as if he was not only convincing me of his decision but also himself. I was losing my ICU overnight partner, but I already had Sean's brother, Joey, lined up to give me some breaks at night.

"I think that sounds like a great plan. Thank you so much for everything you've done so far and being here for me."

"Of course," he responded with a slight smile. I was sad, but so damn proud of him. He was really growing into a wonderful young man and I was so lucky that he even felt comfortable enough to come discuss this with me. He was nervous and unsure, but also knew what he needed to do and I was there to encourage him to do so. My only fear with him returning is that he would have a difficult time focusing on his classes and would feel guilty about not being there with us. After all, he was my child. But I also felt comforted that he had an amazing support system at his school with his fraternity brothers. They were a tight knit group of guys and were always there for one another. He had told me that he was never left alone between the time he got the call from me about Sean and the time that Michael arrived to pick him up in Tennessee. Someone was always sitting with him. Several of the guys even made a trip to the hospital to check in on him and would help get the news out to his professors. Knowing he had that at school, made it a little easier on my mom heart to have him return. He was going to be okay. I was going to be okay.

———

By day eight, Sean was progressing right along and in the right direction. Sara continued to work with him on writing and he was able to write out his name and point to a few pictures when asked to. He was taking more ice chips, drinking out of a straw and then straight from the cup. Physical Therapy got him to stand up briefly with a lot of assistance, but it was still a huge deal. He was completely taken off of oxygen, the a-line that was tracking his blood pressure was taken out, as well as the catheter. He was slowly starting to look a little more human instead of a machine. An IV and feeding tube was all that was left.

As people continued to visit, his urge to talk became even more prevalent. He'd try, but only mumbles and sounds would come out. No words. One of Sean's favorite things to do is talk. He'd rather pick up the phone and talk to someone over texting any day, you just have to have at least an hour available if you saw his name pop up on your phone. There was no such thing as "this will just take a few minutes" with him, no matter how many times he told you or himself that! He enjoyed the connection he could make with people through good ol' fashion conversation. So, stripping his voice from him was complete torture. But I also knew that's what would keep him fighting and not giving up.

Sean started becoming more conscious of things about a week after his stroke. Kathy's pastor from her church showed up to pray over him, as so many others had done before. Kathy, Karen, Landon and myself stood around his hospital bed. He closed his eyes on cue as we all bowed our heads and the pastor said a beautiful prayer, stating his name, and asking for complete healing. When he said 'Amen', I glanced down at Sean and he had tears streaming down his face. He knew it was him that was sick and he was realizing the severity of the situation. We could all see the realization on his face as the tears streamed down our faces to match his. I gave him a reassuring look and whispered, "you're going to be okay." He nodded in agreement as I wiped the tear off his cheek.

Throughout the day, he would greet each visitor with an enthusiastic hug and smile. He really seemed excited to see everyone that would come to visit. That afternoon, during his daily massage from me, I started to get a little more of Sean's personality coming out. The massage led to a little flirting, raising his eyebrows and giving me a crooked grin. I would wink at him and he'd try and wink back. Over the next couple of days, he continued to show me nonverbal love with hand holding and kisses on my hand and forehead. He was coming back. My Sean was coming back to me.

CHAPTER 7

THE UNSEEN WOUND

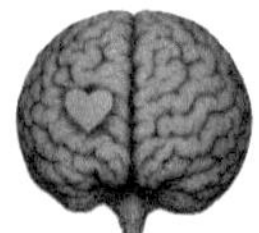

was told many times from the very first day that Sean's stroke recovery would be a lot of "one step forward, two steps back." This wasn't going to be one of those life events that you could put on fast forward no matter how bad you wanted to. In fact, slow motion is more of what the setting was stuck on. Those words held true, but most of the "two steps back" scenarios ended up being more threats.

When he got the ventilator out, his oxygen levels dropped and were staying down. So there was the threat that they would have to put the vent back in. But his levels ended up going up on his own at the last minute. Then came the threat of having to possibly recatheterize him. After having a catheter in for over a week, the bladder muscles naturally weaken and it becomes very difficult to go to the bathroom on your own. But a good, detailed conversation with him of what exactly a recatheterization would entail if he didn't urinate on his own, magically made the pee come out! Sometimes, a good scare tactic works wonders and in this case, it helped that he was beginning to comprehend the words and conversations that we were having with him. Then it was the threat of putting the feeding tube back in. Even though real food and liquids were added back in his diet, they weren't exactly the tastiest foods. Everything was bland and no amount of salt and pepper was going to help. They were worried he wasn't taking in the necessary calories that were required to help build his strength and endurance back up. Especially, when the move to an inpatient rehab facility was literally just days away. If he didn't start taking in more, the feeding tube would be going back in. But extra Ensure protein shakes and ice cream kept the feeding tube from being reintroduced. Overall, he was continuing to move in a forward direction and overcoming all the threats.

I foolishly assumed that the one step forward and two steps back motto applied to all the physical deficits that Sean was experiencing. But in Sean's case the two steps back was his mental health. It was early on day twelve in the ICU when I first started noticing a difference in Sean. Even though I was dealing with my own mental struggles comprehending the heaviness of the situation we were in as a family, I still kept one eye open on Sean for any signs he may start showing. I was warned that depression in stroke patients was very common, and even expected. Not to mention that the area of his brain, the basal ganglia, where he had the bleeding tends to cause depression to come on even faster.

We had just gotten the news that he got the approval to be transferred to inpatient care at Frazier Rehabilitation Institute in Louisville, Kentucky. They are ranked number one in the state of Kentucky and number forty in the U.S. for top rehab hospitals offering state-of-the-art therapies. They have built their reputation as the regional leader in comprehensive acute rehab.*(from Frazier's website) We are extremely lucky to have such a high tech rehab facility right down the road. I was ecstatic that his admission had been approved and we were simply just waiting on a bed to become available. It should have been a day of celebration. But it turned dark pretty fast.

The downside of Sean becoming more aware and his cognitive function returning is that the reality of the situation started sinking in for him. I had noticed the evening before that he was staying asleep for longer periods of time and awake for shorter periods. I chalked it up to his body just needing to rest in order to help heal. After all, sleep was a big part of the healing process as well. But after a full night of good sleep, he woke up the next morning not acting much different. He continued to sleep, refused to eat anything and wouldn't participate in any therapies. The joyful personality that had emerged was quickly shutting down. Like, the door had been slammed shut. He went from hugging and interacting in conversations to just turning everything off, as if someone just flipped the light switch. You would be in the middle of talking to him and he'd turn his head and just close his eyes in mid-sentence. You could physically feel his grieving sadness in the room and it was even more prevalent on his face.

I met Mike and Karen out in the hall outside of his room and mentioned what I had been noticing. To my surprise, they agreed with me and had already been talking amongst themselves about the dramatic changes they were seeing in their son. Now, I knew I wasn't imagining things. I immediately approached every doctor and nurse that came into Sean's room sharing my concerns and demanded something to be done as soon as possible. It was the first time that I felt like I had been taken back to the day I came home from work and found Sean in mid-stroke. And just because it wasn't physical things I was seeing or hearing, I was still watching him decline all over again right before my eyes. Instead of his speech leaving, his face drooping and his body sagging, I was watching his personality leaving, his motivation evaporating and his fight completely disappearing. It was almost scarier to witness.

If he was completely shutting down, how in the world was he supposed to go to an inpatient rehabilitation center the following day and be expected to put in four or five hours of therapy per day? Not only was this going to be physically demanding on his body, but it was definitely going to require the mental state to be on point. And at this moment, his mental state was anything but healthy. The motivation that was going to be required of him to get through the next several weeks, months and even years was just nowhere to be found. There wasn't any amount of pep talks, yelling or begging that I, or anyone else, could do that was going to pick him up out of this funk. The fight was up to him and he was going to have to reach deep down to find that fight in order to survive this curve ball that had been thrown at him. There was simply no other choice. I was desperate for him to find the strength that he needed to fight off this sudden depression.

This wasn't Sean. I had seen him stressed and maybe even a little worried before, but never depressed. Thankfully, it was never an emotion that he experienced. He was always happy and laughing and the life of the party. We had started to see that again, but this damn stroke was stripping that happiness away and replacing it with depression. I was at a loss and felt completely helpless all over again. So what do I do but fall apart myself. The urgency of my begging to the physicians to do something finally caught up with me. At one point I found myself alone in a dark hospital stairwell, hysterically crying. The kind of crying that words can't even come out and you are simply just trying to catch your breath. All I could hear were the tears of my desperation echoing throughout the metal stairwell. I just couldn't pull myself together no matter how hard I tried. I absolutely hated feeling this way.

We were just so fortunate, once again, to have such a caring and attentive medical team working with Sean. Not only were they helping him heal physically, but they heard my cries and noticed as well, the decline of Sean's mental state. Within a few hours, the doctor added an anti-depressant into his already lengthy list of medications he was now taking. I immediately felt a sigh of relief that my concerns were being listened to and taken action on. The mental wound had been bandaged up. Now, I just had to pray that this particular medication would do the trick and bring back the Sean we were seeing just a few days prior.

I never considered the mental side of things as Sean became more aware of the situation he was in. I for sure struggled with everything, as well as the boys, his parents and siblings. We were all coping with what all our new reality was, which was a difficult thing and hard to comprehend, especially when there was zero warning. And our brains were fully functioning. Meanwhile, I couldn't imagine how Sean was dealing with it all with a healing, but injured brain. I played out just about every scenario in my head of where this long road will lead us, went over a million "what ifs" and worried about it all. But then I came across a video of the transformation that Frazier Rehab can do with stroke patients. The video went into detail of how Frazier can physically and cognitively help patients get their lives back together.

Dr. Darryl Kaelin, with Physical Medicine and Neurorehabilitation at the Brain and Spine Institute with Frazier, stated in the video, "We help them (patients) regain their lives with hope and dignity. We create little miracles everyday." He later added "Rehabilitation happens in two stages. Early rehab is about teaching people to compensate for what they have lost. But over the long run, over weeks and months you want them to regain what they have lost." Could they also do this miracle work with Sean, I wondered. One of the stroke survivors, Steve, who was interviewed in the video said, "the doctors at the hospital, they were the ones that saved my life. But the rehab folks are the ones that put it back together." Yes, they can help Sean. I just knew it!

The video sparked not just tears, but hope. Hope that he would say "I love you" again. Hope that he could squeeze my hand with his right hand. Hope that he'll get full function back in his right leg. Hope that he'll be having his daily morning coffee chats with his friend. Hope that he can stand long enough to slow dance with me. Hope he can go to another Nascar race with Mike and Ricky.

Hope that he can do his secret handshake that he only does with Austin every night before bed. Hope that he can talk baseball and attend a game with Landon. Hope that he can drive to the store, work a job he loves and regain his independence. Hope that he can make a full recovery. HOPE!

CHAPTER 8

OUR TEMPORARY HOME

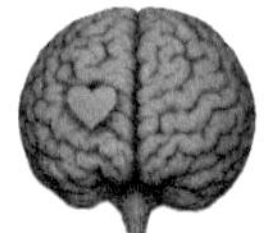

Around 3 p.m. that Wednesday afternoon, and we were anxiously awaiting for the ambulance to arrive to transport Sean from the ICU to Frazier Rehabilitation. Due to safety concerns, we were unable to take him ourselves so we were at the mercy of outside transportation. Since we were scheduled to be discharged that afternoon, all visitors coming to see Sean were gone by noon. Mike and Karen stayed and waited with me to help with the transition over to the new facility. We waited an extra day for a bed to become available but it was finally time to make the move. Although we were ready and excited to be out of the ICU, it was also what we grew comfortable with over the last 13 days. Now, it was time to move forward and learn to be comfortable with our new home. We were finally going to get to see what all the hype was about with Frazier.

Sean was still dealing with his onset depression and had very low energy all day. He continued to sleep more than usual and participated very little, if at all, in conversations and therapies. I became increasingly worried about his mental state but was hopeful that the move out of the ICU would maybe increase his spirits. Sometimes a change of scenery could work wonders. I know I was looking forward to a different four walls to look at. Maybe ones with not so many machines and constant beeping. Three o'clock turned to four, which then turned to five and six o'clock and we still sat waiting at U of L Hospital. I was hungry, tired and becoming extremely anxious. Once again, the feeling of helplessness crept back in and I could feel a cry building up from my gut.

At a little after 7 p.m., EMS finally showed up to transfer Sean. I gathered up our belongings that I could take with me on the ambulance ride with Sean, while Mike and Karen took the rest in their car to meet us over there. Of course there was only one elevator in working order that we could take, so the already long day of waiting around was now spent waiting at the entrance of the elevator, hoping that when the doors opened up there would be no one inside already. We waited and waited and waited, growing more impatient and exhausted each time the door would open and be full of other patients and staff. During that time, I stood next to Sean's side holding his hand. I was nervous for what was to come. I silently said a prayer for peace and comfort over the next few days. While my eyes started the familiar stinging sensation, Sean's remained closed for the most part. He was still shut off from reality. Almost thirty minutes passed before an empty elevator arrived.

When we finally arrived at Frazier, it wasn't the welcome committee that we were expecting. Since we arrived much later than scheduled due to no fault of our own, there didn't seem to be many people there. Day shift staff had left for the day, so the smaller staff of night shift were the only ones around. Lights were turned off or dimmed throughout the halls and overall everything was pretty quiet. It was so different from the busyness of the ICU floor. The EMS driver laid Sean's thick medical chart on the nurses station before taking us into his room. Mike and Karen were already there waiting for us. When I walked in and made eye contact with them, we knew exactly what we all were thinking. "What in the hell is going on?" Mike usually always has questions about everything, but even he was speechless at the moment. We were just going through the motions of where we were being guided, not really having any clue of what was next.

The room was large and clean, but felt very empty for the amount of items that were in such a big room. A single neatly made hospital bed was at one end of the room with a small nightstand next to it. One empty IV pole sat behind the bed. On the other side of the room was a closet and desk with a small desk chair. Upon entry was a large private bathroom. It was made to be wheelchair accessible with hand bars, toilet and shower chairs, amongst other random items that I had yet to learn about their purpose. The vision of that made me feel uneasy for some reason. I was told that a cot would be there for myself to sleep in, a nice change from the hard lounger no doubt, but there was nothing.

Karen began to unpack Sean's suitcase with his clothes and toiletries, I'm sure to keep her mind busy from the silence that overtook the room. The dingy hospital gowns and bright colored grippy socks were a thing of the past. I'm sure Sean will feel better getting into his own clothes for the first time in two weeks. A nurse finally walked in, followed by a staff member from the pharmacy department. We didn't get much of a warm greeting, but instead went straight to business with all the questions.

Except the questions weren't being directed to me. They were looking straight at Sean and waiting on his responses. Sean laid there, speechless, of course, not just because he was completely out of it but because he literally still couldn't speak. I interrupted and started answering the questions being asked.

While the nurse was trying to put a blood pressure cuff on his right arm, the one that still doesn't move at all, the pharmacy staff stopped and said, "Why can't he answer the questions? Is he lethargic or something?" When I tell you that instant rage took over my body, I am not exaggerating. *What in the actual hell is going on right now?* I must be in a Twilight Zone of some sort.

"No, he's not lethargic! He's had a stroke! The right side of his body is not functioning at all and he cannot speak words!" *Why didn't they already know this information about Sean prior to him arriving? They knew he was coming today. Am I going crazy? Did I literally miss hours from this day and don't even realize it?* I was mad that I was even questioning myself even though I did have moments of delirium, so it wouldn't have been that surprising if this mishap fell on me. But looking at Mike and Karen confirmed that this time, it wasn't me.

They quickly made a drastic turn in their questioning, did a pre-examination on Sean and left the room. The three of us looked at each other dumbfounded. It was 8:30 p.m. and an announcement came over the intercom that visiting time was quickly approaching and all guests not staying would be required to leave by 9 p.m. I glanced at Mike and Karen, begging them with my eyes not to leave me here alone. I had nowhere to sleep, Sean was out of it and I was stuck with people that didn't know anything about Sean's condition. I missed the ICU and the staff there. I wanted to go back. Those are words I never thought I'd think. Seeing my worry, Mike scurried out the door to ensure that I would, in fact, have a cot to sleep on that night. They said they were working on finding me one and even though in the moment, that wasn't a satisfactory answer, it was at least an answer.

Another countdown came on the intercom, "fifteen minutes until visiting hours are over."

"Five minutes until visiting hours are over."

"We'll stay," Karen said, also with worry on her face." I don't want to leave you alone here."

"You can't stay. They are strict on their visiting rules." I mumbled back, although I really didn't want them to leave. They hesitantly put their coats on and slowly started gathering their things. As soon as their arms wrapped around me, I fell apart. I sobbed desperately on Mike's shoulder, soaking his shirt, and that was it.

Mike stripped his coat back off and firmly stated, "We're not going anywhere. We're staying with you until we know you are alright and settled in." That was what was so great about them. Mike and I will tend to butt heads at times, but I know he'd do anything for me without hesitation. Although he doesn't say "I love you" with his words, I have no doubt that his love for Sean, myself and his family is there and he'd do absolutely anything for us. He saw me hurting, and he wasn't going to leave. I saw the relief on Karen's face too because I knew she didn't really want to leave either. The three of us stood there, crying together and consoling one another, all while Sean laid still in his bed.

"Visiting hours are over. All guests must leave the building." The voice over the intercom turned into a more stern tone. It was time for them to go.

"It's okay. You all can go. I'll be alright." I was trying to not only convince them, but also myself.

Reluctantly, they agreed to leave. "We'll be back in the morning," Karen said, giving me one last hug good-bye. And with that, I saw them walk out of the room, leaving me in that large, quiet, dark room all alone.

Yes, Sean was physically there, but I felt so terribly alone. I sat in the hard, rigid desk chair and let the tears flow once again. I just cried uncontrollably and felt like I was back in that echoing stair-well again. I wanted to pull myself together, but the all around emotional day had just caught up with me and simply took over my body. I felt like I had so much to release. I reached for another Kleenex and glanced over towards Sean's bed. He slowly opened his eyes. I think it was only the second time I saw his eyes all day.

I tried to mutter out the words, "I'm sorry" but I couldn't get it to come out. He slowly waved me over and I went and sat on the edge of his bed. His left arm wrapped around me and he held my hand. He knew I was upset and he comforted me as much as he was capable of doing at that time. I allowed it by laying down and leaning closer towards him. I continued crying into his chest. I yearned so much to be comforted by the same person that was causing me the pain. It was so strange how the same person could take on both of those roles. I just missed him so much. He was there with me, but in a way, he wasn't. I just wanted my Sean back so badly it hurt, and I didn't want to wait to get him back. Selfish, I know, but I didn't care.

His nurse came back in the room and I tucked myself into my own cot. They had finally brought it in and set it up against the far wall by the large windows that overlooked the emergency helicopter pad. That window would end up providing an interesting distraction during our stay. I watched as she cleaned Sean up, a simple task that he was unable to do for himself. The sadness of the situation I was witnessing with my young husband was beyond what tears could even express. His downcast face was filled with embarrassment and humiliation, yet he knew he needed her help. I turned my head towards the window. I didn't want him to see me staring and honestly, I didn't want to see it either. The last thing he needed was an audience, even if it was just me in the room. The whole situation was so much to take in and comprehend. How has so much changed in just two weeks? I closed my eyes and fell asleep rather quickly due to the exhaustion. I remember hoping that when I woke up, the year 2025 would be over. We were barely in the second month of the year, and I was already over it.

I slept in the next morning and was awakened a little after 8 a.m. with someone tapping me on the shoulder, handing me a slip of paper. I peeled my eyes open to see that it was Sean's schedule for the day. Speech therapy was up first at 8:30 a.m. Pity party Erin got some sleep and it was time to get to work. I turned into a drill sergeant, opening up the blinds, turning the lights on and pushing the button on the side of Sean's bed to sit him up. His breakfast had been delivered at some point that morning, and it was sitting over to the side still covered. The hot coffee was now cold and the Ensure protein shake he had grown accustomed to was room temperature. I took the cover off his food and unveiled his breakfast like it was some magic trick.

Sean had never been a morning person, but lucky for me he loved breakfast and he actually seemed ready to eat for the first time in several days. I had twenty minutes to get him up, fed and motivated. I poured the syrup over his small pieces of pancakes and bite sized portions of sausage. I gave him the best pep talk that I could come up with, which was not just for him but for myself. He had back to back therapies from 8:30 a.m. to 3 p.m. with a break for lunch. There was no time for naps or sulking or feeling unmotivated. It was time to focus and work hard.

Today was the beginning of his healing journey at Frazier and it began with being evaluated by all areas; speech, occupational therapy, physical therapy, and psychology. I had been asked multiple times about the outlay of our home. Frazier's therapists and doctors had one major goal during his time as an inpatient. To prepare Sean as best as they could to move around and survive the daily activities of life in his own home.

I was told the night before the Neurorehab physician that had been assigned to Sean. It was Dr. Darryl Kaelin, aka Dr. Famous from the video I saw a few nights before about the transformation that Frazier could do. I felt like we hit the jackpot getting him. He would make rounds every morning to check on Sean's progress and answer any questions we might have. He came in that first morning to meet Sean and do an evaluation on him. His confidence filled the room when he walked in, much like Dr. Queen and Hot Isaac. I was familiar with it and immediately liked him. He went up to Sean, asking him questions and listening to Sean attempt to answer him. As he was talking to him, he examined his whole body, checking his reflexes, especially on the right side and moving around his limbs. He pulled a pen out of his pocket.

"Do you know what this is Sean?" he asked. Sean tried answering and you could vaguely make out the mumbled word "Pen." Dr. Famous moved his pen from side to side and up and down while he instructed Sean to follow it with his eyes only. Sean was cooperating and showing as much energy as he could.

As he concluded his examination, he put his hand on Sean's shoulder, "We're going to get you better, but it's not going to happen overnight." *Ugh, tell me something I didn't already know.* "You've got to put in the work, but we're going to get you up and moving. I have one last thing we're going to do before I head out." Sean and I both gave an inquisitive look.

"I'm going to sing a song and I want you to try and sing along with me. No need to worry. I know you know it. I can't sing, so I need you to help me. Can you do that with me, Sean?" Sean nodded his head in agreement and I proceeded to move behind his wheelchair. I didn't know what was to come and I wanted Sean's focus on Dr. Famous, while not being distracted by me.

He began, "Row, Row, Row your boat, gently down the stream..." My eyes filled with tears. Again, this reality was getting the best of me. I watched the back of Sean's head bob along with the doctor's singing, but didn't hear him make any sounds. He continued, "Merrily, merrily, merrily, merrily, life is but a..."

Dr. Famous paused and with that Sean muttered out "Dream." It was the biggest word I had heard him say so far. The hopeful tears fell from my eyes. It was such a simple song that most of us learned as a small child, but hearing Sean sing along was so significant in that moment and the look on Dr. Famous's face was telling me the same thing.

"Great job Sean. I'll see you again tomorrow morning. You'll be meeting with your therapists team today and we're all going to work together to get you better and make the most of your time here. We'll be in constant contact with one another as well as with the family so we have specific goals and a plan in place." He shook both of our hands and grinned as if he was saying "it's going to be okay." And with that, he was out the door on the way to his next patient.

Speech therapy reported back first. His therapist was no Sara, my Homegirl and his Speech Therapist from U of L, but she was still very sweet and patient. I loved how she would talk TO Sean versus ABOUT him when she was explaining her findings to me. I found that because he was so difficult to understand and communicate with, some people had a hard time knowing what to do or how to go about talking to him. We finally got an official diagnosis of what was going on with his speech. He had severe Aphasia with Apraxia. Sara had mentioned this several days before, but Frazier's speech therapist confirmed Sara's initial thoughts now that a little more progression had occurred.

Aphasia, a common result of a stroke, can make speaking, understanding, reading or writing incredibly difficult. This language disorder affects the ability to speak, understand, read or write — and it affects nearly one in three stroke survivors. I was told that a key point about aphasia is it does not affect the intelligence of a person suffering from it. People with aphasia still think clearly but may struggle to express or understand words. In the ICU, Sara said Sean had Receptive Aphasia along with Expressive Aphasia. Receptive Aphasia is when he can speak fluently but may say things that don't make sense or have trouble understanding language. When he would try and talk, it would come out very mumbled, almost like a minion from the movie *Despicable Me*. You could make out a few things, but for the most part it was just jumbled together words and sounds.

Sean was diagnosed with only Expressive Aphasia once he was at Frazier. Expressive Aphasia meant he had trouble speaking or writing but can often still understand others. This is why when others would talk to him, the conversation could feel very one sided. And his voice. His voice sounded different too. It was like speaking to a different version of him. The slow pace of his speaking paired with the emphasis that he'd put on certain syllables of the words that would come out, just made him not sound like himself.

Sara explained to me that Apraxia of Speech affects the motor planning for speech. Sean knows what he wanted to say, but his brain struggles to coordinate the movements needed to say the words. Speech may come out slow or sound "off." It is not unusual for apraxia to co-occur with aphasia, especially after a stroke. You could tell that Sean knew exactly what he wanted to say and even how to say it, but his brain just wouldn't let the words come out right or recognizable. This is when frustration would really kick in. He would get frustrated when he couldn't get the words out or explain what he was needing, and we would get frustrated that we couldn't understand him without asking him to repeat himself ten times. Usually, he would give up if it took more than three times, which was often.

Occupational Therapy was next to come in with their findings and plan of action. Their focus was to work on Sean's right arm. There was still no movement, except the tiniest of shoulder shrugs. Not only did the therapist want to work on moving that right arm, but simultaneously wanted to teach him how to do everyday tasks with just his left arm, mostly focusing on grooming techniques of washing face, applying deodorant, brushing teeth and hair, and putting on clothes. All of these things were extremely challenging for Sean to complete and we'd often see the frustration kicking back in.

Physical Therapy was next. A petite, muscular young female entered the room and energetically introduced herself. "Hi, I'm Charley. Ready to get to work Sean?" *What was this little thing supposed to do for Sean?* But she was like a large, manly Army Drill Sergeant stuck in a small, girly body that didn't seem to affect her ability at all to get the job done. She moved him around like he weighed only fifty pounds and hoisted Sean in this sling contraption that was attached to the ceiling on wheels. They pulled it over, dropped it down, securely put it under Sean and buckled him in. The next thing I know, he's "riding" around in this sling ten feet off the ground! They guided the mechanism over and safely placed him in his wheelchair. Sean was anything but amused at the situation, but I, on the other hand, was very impressed. I was beginning to see the perks of what Frazier could do and the nightmare from the check in process days prior were starting to escape my memory. They were quickly making up for that not-so-pleasant arrival process.

Charley and her assistant wheeled him down the hall into the state-of-the-art therapy gym that was directly across the hall from Sean's room. They had everything you could imagine in there to help patients with any disability they were facing. Rows of brightly colored multi-sized balls lined a wall. Stationary bikes, treadmills and other equipment were spread throughout the room. Multiple tables, blocks and mirrors were also scattered around. In the adjoining room to the gym were mock set-ups of showers, toilets and steps, no doubt to "practice" on navigating those things with the newly acquired disabilities that Sean and other patients now faced.

Charley started as well with just the basics for Sean; sitting and standing while keeping his balance. A feat that posed to be much harder than expected. Once that was mastered, they would move to locomotor training on the treadmill while in a harness, walking with assistance and taking on stairs. She would allow Sean to rest when needed, but not for long. She was on a mission to get him better and she didn't respond to laziness well. Although she was tough, she was also extremely encouraging, praising Sean for everything that he'd accomplish.

A psychological evaluation was up the next day. Due to Sean's lack of speech, I was asked to sit in on the first session. Dr. Nancy was a little older and spoke slowly and with intention, with much kindness and understanding in her tone. Since brain injury patients were her specialty, she was able to navigate a conversation with Sean despite his communication difficulties. She concurred with the situational depression that he was having and said that it was extremely common. I had noticed that although I didn't view it as depression, he had started showing more emotion since arriving at Frazier. He would cry easily, especially when he'd see people that meant a lot to him or if he was able to accomplish a task that he couldn't just days before. Dr. Nancy said that emotional release from stroke patients were also very common so these reactions were not surprising to her. So, I guess I now had Sean to cry with me.

I had been told multiple times that music is so healing in situations like this. Not only is it therapy within itself, but singing involves using all parts of the brain. It is a full-brain activity, combining left-brain logic and right-brain artistry. That's one reason it's used in therapies for stroke and aphasia patients.

I reached out to Austin's music director, Patrick, at School of Rock Louisville where he attended drum lessons since he was eight years old. I asked if he'd be willing to come to Sean's room on one of his days off from therapies for a little private concert. Sean loves live music and especially loves watching Austin play. He never misses an opportunity to go to one of his gigs or sit around his drum set at home making song requests while he's practicing for an upcoming show. We've both simply been amazed at the natural, raw talent Austin has for drumming and Patrick and The School of Rock have played an integral role in accelerating those musical abilities.

To my delight, Patrick happily agreed and began working on a set list. He came in that weekend with his acoustic guitar and a small drum set for Austin to play along. For ninety minutes, we were all able to escape the reality we were in. During that time, everything felt normal. If you closed your eyes, you could almost picture sitting around a campfire at the lake, eating s'mores and drinking a cold beer.

Patrick put together medleys of country music classics and upbeat sing-along songs. He started singing "How Sweet It Is" by James Taylor. I looked over at Sean, both of us with watery eyes and we were both singing and tapping our foot to the music. I smiled at him and him at me. In that moment I felt so thankful that he was still here. I soaked in the words to that light-hearted song and just glanced around the room making a mental note of that moment. Patrick sang with a large smile on his face, Austin didn't take his eyes off Sean, Karen was behind me dancing around and Mike was videoing the entire concert on his phone with tears of happiness streaming down his face. We were all experiencing a little joy for the first time in weeks. We were experiencing the power of music and it's exactly what we all needed.

———

We all had survived the first week at Frazier and we were getting adjusted to the more intense schedule. Sean seemed to be participating in everything without push back and we were moving along. Since we had gotten the cot, I was even able to sleep at home more often since Joey, Mike and Karen were in rotation of who was staying with Sean at night. We had our first family meeting with Dr. Famous and the care team. They were happy with his progress so far but there were still many more things they wanted to see him accomplish before he got discharged. Our tentative discharge date was February 28th, which would make for a total of three and a half weeks for inpatient rehab.

It seemed too soon to me for all the things that still needed to be accomplished, but they were the experts. Maybe they saw something that I didn't. We got a little more of a "timeline" of what to expect even though each case can be different. Dr. Famous said that the right leg will probably show movement first, followed by the right arm and then speech is usually the last to return. We should see continued improvement for three to six months, then slower improvement during months six through twelve and speech could take up to two years to come all the way back. He will probably have permanent deficits of some sort with right side movement, even if it is slight. Swelling in the brain still won't be down until up to eight weeks from the date of his stroke. They seemed hopeful overall, but did say to expect that Sean would need 24/7 care for a while once he is home.

After receiving the good report, I felt a little better about the thought of returning to work. We were approaching three weeks since his stroke, and I had yet to go back to work, which meant I wasn't bringing in any money. The stress of the finances was starting to really come to the forefront of my mind. I knew we couldn't afford for me to just stay with him everyday, even though my heart was telling me that was my only option. My mind was beginning to think somewhat clearly again and it was telling me it was time to start reintroducing some work days in the mix of days spent at the hospitals.

It was a Tuesday so I reached out to my boss, Laura, and told her I planned to come back that Thursday and Friday. Maybe just returning for two days would be a good start and then we could go from there. Luckily, Laura was super supportive as well as my loyal massage guests, so I was given the flexibility to come in whenever the days would allow and we could just take things week by week on what my work schedule would look like. Sean continued to attend therapies throughout the day so he was in good hands. He started to say some small words in speech including "yes," "no," "hi," and "go." He was also able to write my name and his name on a white board. Physical Therapy got him up and walking with a harness around him while holding on to rails. Simultaneously, Charley scooted along beside him on a rolling chair and physically picked up the right foot to move it along. They also worked on him being able to maneuver himself around in the wheelchair.

It was my turn to stay the night with him, plus with me going back to work, I would be home the next couple of nights. I nestled under the covers in my little cot and pulled out my journal to start jotting down some thoughts. I heard a rustling noise coming from Sean's bed and glanced over to check on him. He seemed to be having trouble navigating the bed remote. I got up to come over and help him. I took advantage of his alertness after settling on a TV channel that he was satisfied with.

"Can you say, 'Thank You?'" I asked. He grinned back at me with that new, crooked smile.

"Thank…" I paused.

"You." Sean mumbled. I stood there in shock. Did I hear a word?! I tried again to make sure it wasn't a coincidence.

"I love…," once again I paused.

"You." He said again, a bit clearer this time. I began clapping and jumping up and down like an idiot! It was such a small thing but such a big victory in that moment. I was elated. We celebrated with a kiss, I tucked him back in and bounced back over to my cot. No sooner than I got settled back in, he was grunting and causing another commotion. When I walked back over to check on him, he was staring at me with such focus and grit.

"What is it? Are you ok?" I asked. I could tell he wanted to talk so bad.

With much determination, the sounds started coming out. "Good-night" followed up with an "I love you." *Could my ears be deceiving me? Am I going delirious again? Surely, that's not what he was saying.* I had him repeat himself for good measure, several times. The words were mushed together in that minion language. So I repeated back to him, more asking him versus just saying the words.

"Good-night? I love you?" I questioned. He smiled, nodded his head and pointed at me with excitement to confirm that I was guessing his words right. Wow, what a way to end the day! There was so much progression in the last 24 hours. If you would have asked me days before that he'd be telling me he loved me, I never would have believed it. And even though the words weren't clear or spoken at a normal pace, and I had to try several times to guess the words, it was better than anything else I had seen so far. I'd take a mumbled "I love you" any day.

The mental high that I went to bed with the night before came crashing down the next morning with absolutely zero warning. There was no slowing down or even an abrupt stop. It was a full on crash. The morning started out normally with his breakfast being served followed by the little slip of paper with his daily schedule on it. When I approached Sean to get him up, he was sitting in the bed crying. What in the world was going on? I started asking the guessing game questions, trying to figure out if he was in pain or something was wrong. Since there was no chance of him talking to tell me what was going on, I pulled out a picture page that the speech therapist had given him as a helpful tool to communicate with. I pointed to the "pain" picture. He shook his head no, but continued to cry and clearly was upset. I pointed to the "headache" picture and once again he shook his head no.

After going through all the pictures, he said yes to "dizzy" and "nauseous." But something just didn't feel right and my wife's instincts were telling me that physically he was probably okay. The crying turned into lethargy and sitting there completely out of it.

We got him moved to a chair to attempt going to Occupational Therapy, but he began to slump over, looking as if he was going to fall right out of the chair as he was barely even keeping his eyes open. This scene felt all too familiar as the one in the ICU. He was going into a mental funk again. I took it upon myself to reach out to Dr. Nancy, his psychologist. I wanted him to be seen as soon as possible. Meanwhile, the medical staff went into panic mode, ordering a CT, lab work, urine analysis and checking all of his vitals. No medications had changed, so they needed to figure out the root to Sean's quick change of mood and attitude.

By 11 a.m., I was back to being an emotional mess. Talk about an emotional roller coaster. I was feeling elated just 12 hours earlier and now was back to uncontrollable fear and worry. Sean continued to sleep and was showing no emotion for the short periods he'd open up his eyes.

The medical imaging technicians entered the room. "Mr. Troklus, we're ready to take you down for your CT." Although my gut was telling me this was his depression kicking back in, I was thankful that the staff wanted to rule out any other issues and they were taking urgent steps to do so. No one else had arrived yet that day, so there I was again by myself in the large room as I watched Sean being rolled out and taken down the hall to the medical imaging department. I was stuck there with nothing but my thoughts and worries. It was literally one of the worst places to be.

Over the intercom in a loud, monotone voice, I heard, "Code Blue, Frazier Rehab, CT. Code Blue, Frazier Rehab, CT. Code Blue, Frazier Rehab, CT." Pure panic raced through my veins.

Sitting on the side of my cot, rocking back and forth and muttering prayers out loud, I picked up my phone and opened the Google search bar. I frantically searched, "What does Code Blue mean?" It was the first time since Sean's stroke that I did a Google search of any kind. I knew looking up any of his symptoms or diagnoses would only put me in a tail spin and do absolutely nothing for my mental health. But in this case, I was desperate and alone. Sean had been gone for around five minutes at that point so the probability that this code was for him was very high.

The results popped up immediately from my search. "A 'code blue' in a hospital is an emergency code indicating a patient needs immediate medical attention, usually due to cardiac or respiratory arrest." I immediately regretted my decision to consult with Google. I was thrown into hysterics and I wasn't just asking God to spare Sean, I was begging Him. My instinct must have been wrong and something really was physically wrong with him. I clutched his wedding band that was still on my necklace and squeezed my eyes shut, continuing to pray that Sean would return to me. It was a long ten minutes to be alone.

By 11:20 a.m. they were wheeling him back in. Not a word was said to me. I sat dumbfounded at his return, but also extremely gracious. My begging prayers had worked. Although Sean was still in a lethargic state and he remained still with his eyes closed, it was clear at that time that the Code Blue was not about him. The sigh of relief only led to the release of grateful tears on my part.

All the tests being conducted continued to come back normal. All vitals were where they wanted them to be, urinalysis looked awesome and CT results came back unchanged from the CT scan two weeks prior. The day had been so emotionally draining and the original thought of returning to work the next day was no longer an option. I wasn't leaving Sean after this day. He had only been awake maybe thirty minutes the entire day and we still didn't have a definitive answer as to why he was acting the way he was. It would be another night for me on the cot.

The following morning was like the day before never happened. Sean picked up right where he left off two days before. He ate a good breakfast, interacted with me and was ready for his day of therapies. *How often was this roller coaster of emotions going to occur?* I don't think I can handle this on a regular basis. There was only so much I could take. Dr. Famous visited that morning and confirmed that all the test results coming back were not showing anything, he agreed that more than likely it was all related to his acute depression.

So, I was right. Never doubt a wife's instincts. Dr. Famous once again confirmed that the chemical imbalance of where the bleed was tends to cause depression much quicker. "You know him best and we do take your opinions into consideration, but we had to make sure there weren't any new underlying issues." It did make me feel better that my concerns were being listened to and even validated.

Laura Watkins, my boss, who also happens to be the author of a memoir about mental health called "Something Feels Off: Thriving in Life & Business Beyond a Mental Health Crisis" explained to me that the brain chemistry became imbalanced from all the other things going on with Sean's brain injury. There's been an interruption in the "wiring of his brain" so to speak, so the chemicals can't flow naturally through the neurotransmitters to keep everything balanced. This may explain why it comes on so suddenly and then the next day it's better.

The "one step forward and two steps back" continued over the next week. Valentine's Day fell on that Friday and was also my first day going back to work. I made it through three of the four massages. My last massage guest asked one too many questions about Sean and the tears started flowing. I knew if I got started, I couldn't stop so I kept my composure all day up until that moment. At that point, all I wanted to do was get back to Frazier to check on him.

Ricky brought in balloons and chocolates for me from Sean and when I walked in the room, he greeted me with a smile and the attempt to say "Happy Valentine's Day," a difficult phrase for him to say. He was sitting up in his bed holding a card. I opened it. Inside, he wrote "Smitty loves Sean."

I wasn't sure who Smitty was, but I guessed it was me! He was so proud of himself, so I wasn't about to question who and where "Smitty" came from. He could call me Smitty anytime he wanted.

It was a one step forward moment. All six of my Homegirls showed up that evening to visit Sean and kidnap me to take me to dinner. They promised to have me back in time for dessert with my Valentine. It was a sweet gesture and I know they just wanted to get me out of a hospital setting, but I really wanted to just stay with Sean. I already felt guilty returning to work that day instead of being there with him.

Earlier that same day, the dietitian came in with concerns about Sean's eating habits. He wasn't drinking and eating enough to keep up the strength that his therapies demanded. She planned to speak to Dr. Famous about maybe changing around his medications. In the meantime, whoever was staying with him, were required to write down everything he consumed over the next few days so they could evaluate it on Monday. If things didn't improve over the weekend, a feeding tube would have to go back in. Two steps back.

The magic dish that would keep the feeding tube from going back in? Cheesecake Factory's Fresh Strawberry Cheesecake. Kelly brought us up a few pieces for Valentine's Day and he gave no push back on eating it. It was like the food that opened up his stomach to be willing to eat more. So, we were able to dodge the feeding tube bullet. One step forward.

Then we started to deal with some of the changes in his medication. There was so much tone on his right side from not being able to move, that a high dose of a muscle relaxer was prescribed. Well, it helped with the tone (one step forward), but made him very tired. He was unable to participate in his therapies and couldn't give the full participation needed to get results. So, it took a while to get the dosage adjusted to the correct amount. Two steps back.

At the weekly family meeting with Dr. Famous, he said he was very happy with his progress and he was pretty much moving in a forward direction. This upcoming week's plan was to focus on bladder training and continue working on walking and going up steps. For the family, they wanted to put us through a training session on proper and safe ways to move Sean and transfer him around. He was no longer using the sling attached to the ceiling but instead, nurses and aides would come in and move him using a Gait Transfer Belt. Mike and I decided that we would be the ones to go through the training. Since I would be alone with him and doing the majority of the caregiving, I was an obvious choice, but on the days I'd be at work or taking care of business, it would probably be Mike, with Karen or Kathy. Sean still depended on someone 100% of the time to do anything, and his discharge date of February 28th was rapidly approaching.

I continued to go to work a couple of times a week and was building up my tolerance and my emotions to get through full days. Whoever was staying with him during the day at Frazier, were constantly keeping me updated so I was never not in the know of what was going on. I'd leave work and drive straight to Frazier to be with him either for the night, or until the voice came on the intercom to tell me that visiting hours were over.

With just one week to go before discharge, I had my caregiver training with Sean and the physical therapist. They really focused on the proper techniques to transfer him from the bed to the wheelchair and then from the wheelchair to the car. They had a full sized car in one of their gyms so I was really able to get an idea of what that would be like in real life. And let me tell you, it was much harder than I thought it would be. I thought I was going to waltz in there and just sling him around with no problems. After all, that was what the therapists looked like when they did it. I was put in my place real quick. Instead of easy, the transfers were extremely awkward and I struggled with it. A lot. There were so many "rules" to follow. Pick him up this way, hold your body this way, hold his body that way, keep his right knee locked so it doesn't buckle, move your feet like this, don't go this direction… oh, and don't drop him. I felt like I was doing everything wrong and was very overwhelmed by the end of the training. They gave me a yellow band to keep on hand showing that I had completed the training, but I definitely didn't feel like I deserved it. I was far from ready in my opinion. I was going to need a lot more help before I felt comfortable with safely moving him.

Over the last week there, I continued to come in for extra training with whoever was willing to help. I got a lesson on taking him to the bathroom and giving him a shower and doing transfer after transfer after transfer. Although I was feeling a little better about things, I grew increasingly anxious as the discharge date approached. He wasn't ready to come home yet. I wasn't ready for him to come home yet. The move was very scary. Just like when we left the ICU, we became dependent on all the medical staff that was there 24/7 to help with his care. *How was I going to do this without them?* I started mentioning my concerns to the therapists, doctor and case manager. I wanted him to stay longer. I was hoping that me speaking up would keep him at Frazier. What started out as a not great experience upon arrival, turned into a place that definitely lived up to their hype. They were so good at their jobs and helping with Sean's recovery, I didn't even want him to leave! I just wanted to take everyone home with us. To my disappointment, my requests for him to stay longer was denied. He was going home.

———

I stayed with Sean the night before his discharge. We woke up the next morning full of anxiety. Even though Sean wasn't talking, I could tell he felt the same way as I did. I tried staying upbeat and positive about the move, but on the inside, I was terrified. The morning was chaotic. When Sean woke up, I went over to remove the leg brace that he had to sleep in every night. I slung it around like I usually did, and he let out a painful yelp! Wait a minute, this was his right leg!

"Did you just feel that?" I exclaimed. He nodded his head yes with aggression. YOU'VE GOT TO BE KIDDING ME! We're scheduled to go home within hours and he was going to start getting feeling back? I got the nurse immediately and she came in for a quick examination. Sure enough, with the slightest move, he'd grimace in pain. They called the doctor in. It was explained to us that as the nerves start "waking up," it can send sensations of pain to the brain, even though in reality, there is no pain being experienced. A nerve medication would now be added to the long lists of medications that he was now on.

Kathy and Ricky showed up to help with the transition home, while Mike and Karen got the house ready for our arrival that afternoon. After the doctor left, the pharmacy tech showed up with a bag full of sixteen medications that were to go home with us. A medical equipment company walked in and dropped off a new wheelchair and bedside commode. The nurse came in to go over all of the discharge instructions and dos and don'ts once getting home. Print name here, initial here, credit card please and signature required. It was one paper after another. Sean sat in the wheelchair watching as I was spinning from one side of the room to the other, the chaos of being pulled in every direction kept me from crying. Ricky and Kathy began gathering up all of our belongings and stuffing the bags with the extra briefs, gloves, sanitary wipes and other items that we had in the closet. Everything was packed up and we had put off the good-bye long enough.

Ricky and Kathy left to load up the cars and bring my car around to the front of Frazier to pick us up. My responsibility at that point was gathering up Sean. He was safely secured in the wheelchair and I started to wheel him out of what had been our temporary home for the last four weeks. It was coming to an abrupt end.

Nurses, therapists and other staff lined the halls as we exited our room and the floor. We were being escorted out with applause, hugs and well wishes. When we got to the elevator, I didn't want to push the button and even hesitated doing so. I looked over at Sean and he was crying. That's all I needed to get my tears flowing. We were both scared and it was showing on our faces.

I used the techniques I learned and safely got him loaded into my car. I folded up the wheelchair and hoisted it into the back. I hopped in the driver seat, looked at Sean and took a deep breath. "Ready or not, here we go," I muttered under my breath but making it loud enough for Sean to hear me. I grabbed a hold of his left hand and he squeezed it back. I put the car in drive and saw Frazier Rehabilitation moving further away in my rearview mirror. The radio had been turned off and there were no words spoken on the 25 minute drive home, only silent cries from both of us. We were driving into the unknown and it was up to me to make sure we were going to survive this transition. I pulled in the driveway. I looked at Sean with watery eyes and he looked back at me. Simultaneously, we took another deep breath. Here goes nothing.

PART TWO
NAVIGATING THE UNKNOWN

Through Every Step

By Yvonne Kent Pateras

They say love is easy when the road is smooth.
But real love, the kind that holds is tested when the
    path is steep.

It's in the long hospital corridors.
The slow mornings.
The thousand little tasks that used to take seconds,
    now done with patience and care.

It's the hand that never lets go -
Not out of duty,
But because it wants to be there.

Disability may change the pace,
But it cannot dim the bond of two people

Who choose, every day,
To walk or roll side by side.

There will be days of frustration,
Moments of doubt,
And nights where the weight feels too heavy.

But there will also be laughter in unexpected places,
Small victories worth celebrating,
And a deeper knowing:
That this love has roots deeper than hardship can
     reach.

True love is not measured by perfection,
But by persistence.
By showing up.
By saying,
"We are still us…and we are still here."

Because together,
Every obstacle becomes another step
On the journey they promised to take -
Hand in hand,
Through every season,
Through every step.

CHAPTER 9

RINSE AND REPEAT

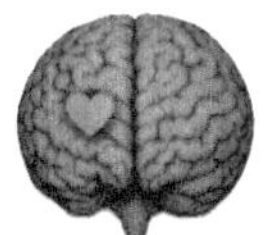

found out within the first day that I was never going to be able to keep up with all of the medical information being thrown my way. It was in-depth, mostly medical jargon and it was a lot. I was being greeted around every corner with a new specialty physician or nurse or therapist that approached me with a wealth of information and updates on Sean's status. This was also coming at me when I am not thinking clearly and having troubles keeping my own thoughts together without new info taking up the little space in my brain I had left.

I immediately opened up my phone and began taking notes. I wrote down everything. I mean everything. Doctor's names, medications being added and taken away, tests being conducted and why, results of said tests, time a bath was given or teeth brushed, when he opened his eyes for the first time and when he mumbled his first word. And everything was stamped with a date and time. I didn't want to miss a single piece of information that was being thrown my way.

It was also a way to remember how far he was moving forward and improving with time. When you're living in the day to day of stroke life, things become very slow and your patience is tested in every way. You feel at times that nothing is happening and time is standing still. But when I'd look back at my written notes, and even pictures and videos that I would document along the way, I was shocked to see how much progress he was actually making. And even more importantly, Sean could see where he started and how far he'd come .

My original intentions for the note taking were to keep my facts straight and to be able to relay accurate information to family and friends looking for Sean updates. As I continued typing them out every day, I changed up my wording and wrote the notes out as if it was an update TO Sean versus just ABOUT Sean. Not only did this keep me in a positive mindset with hopes he will one day be able to read again, but also added a personal touch to the notes. The doctors told me that he probably wouldn't remember anything about his time in the ICU, so it was up to me to write out his progress and setbacks and accomplishments so that he could have it to read when he was ready. He could read his story of being a stroke survivor.

I wanted to also have an outlet for myself where I could journal the emotional side of the stroke journey. If this is your reality, I promise that you feel every emotion known to man. Every high and every low will punch you in the gut and you'll feel its aftermath at your core. I needed a way to release those emotions, not just through tears. I needed to heal through writing, as well. I was learning to do that by putting my pen to paper, something that was very out of the ordinary for me. Plus, I didn't want to burden my friends and family, so writing it all down was my best option. The majority of my personal journal entries have been transcribed word for word in this chapter. They're exactly what I was feeling and going through in those moments.

———

Overwhelmed, I opened the new journal that my Homegirls gave me. It's the only word that came to mind to write down on the first blank page. We were five days into Sean's stroke journey and it was still the top emotion I felt since day one. I had never been big on journaling. I tried multiple times but never stuck with it and always had an excuse for quitting. But I knew that journaling now was not only important, but necessary for me to keep my emotions in check and my thoughts in order. It was my "Emotion Journal" of sorts. I took a deep breath and let the pen flow on the paper.

"Overwhelmed. Most things have been a complete blur between now and five days ago. I, myself, feel like I'm in and out of consciousness. Is this my reality or just a complete nightmare? It's both - a nightmare that has become real life. We have had such an outpouring of love and support, that I literally can't keep up with it all. I have to wait until I'm going to sleep at night before I can even read all the texts, comments and cards from everyone sending their thoughts and prayers. I'm hearing from not just our close family and friends, but from old co-workers, extended family, my massage guests, friends from the past and even from people I've never heard of.

Pastors are coming in and praying over Sean's body. Our closest friends have pretty much stepped up to a level of friendship that I didn't even know was possible! It's overwhelming. We are having food brought to us and goody bags with books, blankets, overnight items and cash donations to get me and the boys through this nightmare. Life, as we knew it, has just halted. Overwhelming! Landon is home from school and I'm not going to work because we don't want to leave Sean's side. I'm not the only one in and out of consciousness. So is Sean. He's making progress one minute and scaring us the next.

The doctors say this will probably be at least a year recovery. Overwhelming. I'm pretty sure I've gone through every emotion possible - scared, worried, mad, elated, tired, stressed, thankful. Rinse and repeat. Rinse and repeat. Rinse and repeat."

I look over and see the box of tissues laying where Sean should be. Landon was staying with him tonight so I could come home. Writing down my thoughts did make me feel a little less lonely but it was still cold in our king bed without him in it. I grabbed one of the tissues and continued writing.

"Scared. There have been a few times in my life where I truly felt scared, but this I have to say, was the most scared feeling I've ever had! January 24th coming home from work with Sean in the middle of a stroke. I watched Sean leave me before my very eyes, scared to death that he would never return to me. I thought I was losing him. The hours and days to follow were just continued feelings of panic and being scared. I'm being told by the doctors that he'll be lucky to fully recover without deficits of any kind. Scared. How are we going to get through this year with one son in college, Sean now without a job and me not being able to work because I want to be there for him?!

Scared. Oh, and being told 'It's a marathon, not a race,' 'be patient,' and 'it's all unknown.'

Unknown. That's a word that I don't handle well. I am a very Type A personality. I am very organized, and I plan my life out months and even years in advance. I'm the opposite of a procrastinator and don't understand how anyone can function through life waiting until the last minute to complete a task. I save, I research, and I make checklists. Actually, I thrive on a good checklist. Nothing is more satisfactory to me than being able to check something off a long list of to-do items. I am meticulous with details and will read every review before purchasing an item or booking a vacation spot. I am a rule follower and think in black and white. I don't do any shades of gray, and I don't do "unknown."

I'm convinced that God was testing every one of my personality weaknesses with Sean's stroke. Everything about his condition is unknown. And I'm just trying to figure out how to accept that new word into my vocabulary, especially when it comes to the question "when will I ever get my husband back?"

The exhaustion was taking over my body and I was feeling heavy all over. I closed up my journal for the night. I released enough for the day. I no doubt had plenty to still write about. When I opened up my journal the following night, I decided to change my wording and write the journal entries like letters to Sean. I continued where I left off from the night before.

"Worried. After being scared, it all turned to worry. Worry if you're going to be able to move again, worry if and when you're going to talk again, worry if your personality will be different as you become more alert.

After all, your brain is bleeding! Are you going to recognize and know me, your sons, parents, friends and family? You have eased that a little as the days go by. On day five, I got a purposeful hug from you. It was the hug we both needed. In that moment, you knew who I was.

You knew I was your wife and best friend."

I began crying. I looked over from my hard lounger in the small hospital room and watched Sean sleep. His body was tired, and his brain was injured. It was absolutely heartbreaking seeing him in this state and struggling to put the pieces together. He's trying to understand what happened and why he doesn't feel like himself. I continued writing.

"Worry. I worry about the frustration that you are going through and will continue to go through in the upcoming days, months and years as you start rehab and therapies and when you realize that you can't do the everyday things that you're used to doing. I worry about if God is going to give you, me, the boys, your parents and family the patience that is going to be required to get us through this challenging time that we are having to face head on. I have faith He will, but I think we will be tested for sure. Then comes the financial side of things.

Talk about worry! You're going to lose your job. It's almost a given. There's no way they can hold your position for you for a year or more. And that's even assuming that you can do the same type of work. With no job, comes loss of benefits and health insurance. What do I do then?! And I need to be here to help you, so how do I go back to work? I know I'll have to go back at some point - we can't go a year with neither of us working. Bills don't stop just because of tragedy, which is what this is.

Another big worry is the boys. Landon has been so great, but I've watched him struggle, especially the first several days. I know he is debating on what to do about returning to school. Selfishly, I want him to stay because his calming presence always soothes me. But I know he needs to return to school and that is what I am encouraging him to do. Then there is Austin. I'm worried about him because I think he's the only one I haven't seen cry. I check in with him and he always responds with 'I'm fine.'

Maybe he cries when he was alone at night. Lord knows, that's what I'm doing.

I'm just so concerned he was just holding everything in, and I know that isn't healthy. I'm trying my best but feel like I'm failing him by not being there the way a mom should be there to comfort their child. He has maintained his daily schedule going back to school immediately. I think maintaining some normalcy was good for him to help cope with what was going on. He's only coming up to the hospital every few days to visit. I don't want to pressure him to come up, but instead visit when he's ready.

The good news is he is able to see a more drastic change in your recovery, versus the rest of us who are here on the daily. And when he returns to the hospital, I know he's been thinking on things because he will drill the doctors with questions!"

It had been several days since I opened up my journal, and it seemed as if so many things were happening so quickly with Sean's progress, therefore sitting down to write just didn't fit into the schedule. "Elated," I jotted at the top of the page.

"Elated. One of the good emotions that I've experienced throughout this experience. For the most part, starting around day three or four, you're showing lots of progress and very few, if any, setbacks. So elation is coming regularly as there was something new to celebrate each day as you continued to show baby steps of improvement. We can literally see the prayers being answered right before our eyes.

I'm praying for continued recovery and thanking God for what He's done up to this point. I'm literally witnessing miracles. I went from thinking I was going to lose you to preparing for the move to inpatient rehab. You no longer need the ICU! I'm also elated about the care team you had while in the ICU. All the staff were so amazing. Dr. Queen and Dr. Leanhardt, Hot Isaac and your nurses and therapists. They were all so compassionate towards you and the rest of us.

That was the team that made you better, but rehab is where you will start getting your life back. We're all elated."

I decided to end my journal entry on a high note. I put my pen away and shut the spiral bound book. The once-empty journal was starting to fill up with more of my emotions, but now the back of the book was filled with doctor's notes and medications and my favorite, to-do checklists. And there were a lot of them. I was slowly starting to take some of the business-related responsibilities, or at least attempting to. I still hadn't returned to work at this point, but knew the day would have to be coming soon.

I was tired. Considering I felt this word to my core, it was a no-brainer to write about it.

"Tired. Oh my, has this whole thing been so tiring. My body is tired. My mind is tired. I'm getting broken sleep, continuing to alternate one night at the hospital and the other one at home. The papers, forms, texts, applications are being thrown at me 24/7 and it is impossible to keep up with it all, especially when I only want to ignore it and just sit by your side.

And when I think about how tired I am, I can only imagine how tired you are. It's about a week in when you started to become more aware of what's going on. I was told to try to tell you what happened. So, you've been in a medically induced coma, woken up in a strange place and told you've had a stroke. All while your brain is still very injured and swollen. Even though we've moved to Frazier Rehabilitation, you're still being woken up non-stop for round-the-clock medications. You are so tired.

You're sleeping a lot, which they say is normal with stroke patients. For every fifteen minutes of physical therapy, you sleep for two hours. And now that you're inpatient, the therapies are a lot more intense so there's less time for naps. It's obvious that you're physically tired, but I could tell mentally, you're just exhausted. You get frustrated very easily. But who wouldn't be when their voice has been stripped from them, and they can't communicate? I think we are all just at the beginning of the tired phase. We may have no idea what tiredness actually is. I just hope we can all get a little rest at some point."

"Stressed. Since Day one, this has been probably the most stressful event I have ever been through. The ups and downs, the highs and lows; it has been the definition of a roller coaster. One day, you are accomplishing so much and moving forward and the next day all you want to do is sleep. You are unmotivated in every way. The heaviness of this whole stroke has left us all stressed beyond anything else we've ever experienced. It has taken a toll on all our mental health. I've never in my life seen you as down and depressed as I've seen you over the last three weeks.

No, it hasn't been everyday. In fact, most days have been good but the few days you have been down, you've been really down. These days not only stress me out, but they scare me to death. I've never felt weaker than in those moments too. I feel helpless, yet all I want to do is help you. Help give you motivation and encouragement. But on those days, you refuse to hear or see anything. I know you are stressed. I can't even imagine what you're going through or what you are thinking and feeling. But the stress isn't going to take us down. I am strong and you are strong. And together, we're going to fight this and come out better on the other side.

I've prayed to God so much the last several weeks. And I pray to take the stress away. Stress and worry go hand-in-hand for the most part so usually if I'm feeling one emotion, I'm feeling the other. I'm not ready for the stress to take me down and I'm not giving up...and I hope you're not either."

I, once again, decided to end my journal entry on a high note. I wrote "thankful."

"Thankful. What an odd feeling to have through all this but I really am. The number one thing I'm thankful for is that you're still here with me. Day one was the worst day ever but I've been holding on to one thing. I was told how lucky you were that I found you when I did. How different things could be at this point, had the stroke happened earlier that morning, or my massage guest was unable to come in earlier, which allowed me to go home sooner than expected. That was the first time I felt thankful. You're going to make it, but not without challenges. I'm going to still have you in my life and that's all that matters. Over the weeks, days, hours and even minutes, I have felt thankfulness.

Even though we are all living a nightmare right now, there is still a lot of hope. You're making baby steps each day and improve in some way. It may be that you're moving a little more or talking a little more or accomplishing a small task. But it mostly is moving in a forward direction and I am very thankful for every bit of that. I am thankful for your progress, your ambition and fight. Simply thankful."

———

I highly recommend keeping your own "Emotion Journal." My intentions were to keep most of these thoughts to myself. They were my thoughts and feelings and that alone. But I want to help others going through a similar situation even more than I do just keeping these thoughts to myself. Express your feelings. Feel every ounce of the pain and the gratitude. Talk about the good, bad and the ugly. Write your story. Your struggles may be someone else's survival guide. You never know who it might help. Or at the very least, how it will help you cope and accept this unimaginable life change.

CHAPTER 10
TRIAL AND ERROR

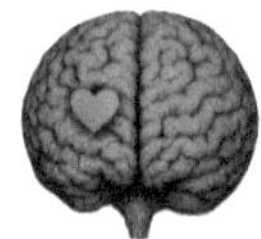

Mike and Karen met us in the driveway when we pulled in from arriving home from Frazier. Melissa's husband was frantically working inside our garage building a wheelchair ramp for Sean. Although Dr. Famous told us we originally weren't going to need a ramp, Charley thought it might be a good idea to have one for a short while until he was further along in outpatient physical therapy. The final decision was made just two days before we came home to install a ramp. Luckily, Melissa's husband was very handy and had already been out to the house to get measurements. By the time we arrived home, an entire ADA compliant wheelchair ramp was almost fully built in our garage. That last minute decision proved to be a wise one.

Ricky and Mike attempted to help Sean up the front porch steps while the ramp was waiting to be completed and it was no simple task. Our steps did not have a handrail of any kind and were much taller than the ones practiced on in therapy. Sean was able to provide very little help while Ricky held him up and Mike tried moving his feet. They were worn out and breathing heavily by the time they got up the three steps into the house. Although Ricky had experience in the nursing field of moving patients around, the rest of us were scared to death that Sean was going to fall. And from the look on Sean's face, he was equally as terrified. So the ramp that I didn't even think was going to be needed ended up being one of the best things to have built and ready. Not to mention all of the multiple appointments that he was going to continue to go to with having to get him not just IN the car but TO the car. Having the ramp saved us so much time and frustration. Trial and error.

During the last week in Frazier, instead of my thoughts and feelings, my journal started to fill up with to-do lists, items to purchase and things to get ready around the house for Sean's arrival home. I had pages of things that I anticipated we would need or would happen and how they would all go down. I was essentially in my nesting phase. You know the phase that occurs around the 8th month of pregnancy when you know you're about to bring a newborn home very soon, so you begin preparing your home for the big change? I had a delivery arriving almost daily and had been getting things out and organized in the areas of the house where I thought they would be the most useful. There was still a stack of unopened Amazon boxes outside our bedroom door that I hadn't even gotten to yet and honestly, I couldn't even remember what was in them. Kathy and Karen began helping me unpack the bags and open up the delivered boxes.

Before unpacking, I was already getting sidetracked with Mike and Ricky settling Sean in. Once they got him in the house, I had his wheelchair from the hospital waiting for him right inside the front door entrance. Needless to say, it was the first time a wheelchair had been in our house. We hit our first roadblock when we moved less than ten feet into the house as we aimed to get him to the couch. The wheelchair wouldn't fit around the front corner where the couch was closest to the TV wall. We turned around to go the other way, yet quickly found out that the wheelchair also struggled to fit between the back of the couch and back wall of the room. The wheels of the chair brushed against the backside of the couch and the arm rests scraped the wall. Well, this clearly wasn't going to work.

Within minutes, we were rearranging the entire living room. The same set-up that we've had for over twenty years was getting a complete makeover, but not the fun kind that you see on the reality TV shows. It was the wheelchair accessible kind of makeover. The couch was pushed flush all the way to the back wall allowing no walkway behind like before. The sofa table and end tables were no longer in their appropriate spots as they were now seen as a line of random tables against the wall at the front of the living room. Deep indentions of all the furniture left their marks in the carpet where they once were. Trial and error.

Getting on the soft cushiony couch, or more importantly, getting up from the couch was going to be nearly impossible for Sean. The seat of the couch sat lower to the ground and sunk down even further when you sat down. This, of course, was never even given a thought prior to getting him home. So the Lazy Boy that was nestled in the far front corner of the room was moved next to the couch that was now set up against the back wall as well. The chair we hardly ever sat in before became Sean's "spot" for the foreseeable future. Trial and error.

Once Sean was finally settled into the Lazy Boy, we first tackled the bathroom. It was quickly filled with organized clutter for anything and everything that Sean might need. A new bathrobe hung on a hook next to the shower with a pair of non-skid slippers lying right under it. A stack of new towels and washcloths laid in a corner of our bathroom closet to use not just for showers but for the anticipated accidental messes that happens when your body is relearning how to function normally. Jill's husband installed a new hand-held shower head suggested by the Occupational Therapist (OT) that was delivered a few days before we got home. I pulled a set of safety shower bars out of a box and suctioned them to the shower walls in the places where I thought would be best and according to how I practiced shower time at Frazier with the OT.

We then assembled the shower bench and placed it inside the shower. We proceeded to all take turns maneuvering the wheelchair to the perfect 90-degree angle to the shower bench, attempting to get in and out of the shower based on how we thought Sean would be transitioned (by me). Again, basing all the locations from my practice rounds at Frazier. After all, we took pictures of the layout of our shower and bathroom specifically for this purpose. I even consulted a video I took during the transitioning process while I was getting my training.

We discussed the placement of the chair and bench for entirely too long and all argued our opinions of what would work best, finally settling on a placement we could all agree on. Meanwhile, Sean sat alone in the Lazy Boy in the living room where we left him with the TV remote nearby. Also something he had to relearn how to use.

In front of the shower bench I rolled out and laid a non-skid mat to keep from slipping when being transferred. I knew shower time was going to be one of the biggest challenges, but it wasn't going to be because of a lack of preparation on my part.

The first shower at home was, for lack of a better word, interesting. Since I was the only one doing shower duty, an obvious job for the wife, I was completely on my own for this process. Mike sat outside the bathroom door anxiously awaiting a yell of help if I were to need him. Luckily, we do have a good sized walk-in shower that allows just enough room for the shower bench, Sean and then me in the front.

It was a tight squeeze but Sean was determined to get all the way inside so that the shower door could shut all the way. Originally, the bench was set up to be halfway in the shower and halfway out. So, all of the discussions and arguing over where the best place for the bench to sit was for nothing. I also didn't take into consideration that I would be in the shower with him the whole time to help with everything. Sean reached out multiple times as well for the grab bars, but he was reaching where I didn't have them installed. Well, those will have to be moved. Trial and error.

I found myself literally spinning in a tight circle up front, holding the hand-held shower head while the cord would wrap around me when I'd reach for a shampoo bottle, pick up a wash cloth on the floor, help him lift his right arm, attempt to help him stand, wash him, wash myself and spin around some more. After the showering was complete, then I had to work on getting him out. I got out first, drying off and getting my clothes on and some non-skid shoes myself. The last thing I needed was to slip while picking him up.

The bathrobe was a process to get on him, especially his right arm since it was not only immobile, but also had developed a lot of spasticity. This caused his arm and hand to bend due to the increase in muscle tone. Even with this challenge, he insisted on wearing it. Time to move him from the shower to his wheelchair. I positioned him, I positioned myself and I positioned the wheelchair. I got what I thought was a good hold on him.

"One, two, three!" we counted out loud together. He went up, I lost my grip and immediately he went right back down with only half of his body landing back on the bench. The other half hanging off the front and me tangled up next to him, praying he wasn't going to fall all the way to the floor. I let out a yelp.

Mike immediately yelled, "Everything okay?"

"Yes!" It kind of wasn't okay, but I was determined to complete this task on my own. I wasn't going to have Mike or anyone else be around for every future shower!

I managed to maneuver ourselves around and got him up and safely to his wheelchair. My heart was racing and I'm sure Sean's was too. I got him dried off and dressed. The whole shower process was exhausting and literally took a massive amount of energy on Sean's part. I even found myself getting a good workout with all of the moving around and transitioning required. Mike sat outside the bathroom door waiting for the first shower process to be completed for one hour and fifteen minutes. Trial and error occurring the entire time.

Trial and error occurred over the next several showers. We tweaked things each time finding something small that would make things just a little easier for both of us, each shower decreasing the time by a few minutes. Maybe it would be the process of putting on his robe or the way we'd position the wheelchair outside of the shower door or the order in which the clothes come off or go on.

Also, over time, he gained a little more strength and got a little more movement to assist me in assisting him. One year later, we now have shower time down to fifteen minutes flat. Twelve minutes on a really good day. But it took a lot of trial and error.

The bathrobe and slippers, on the other hand, were a hit with Sean. It was perfect to keep him warm (it was March and still chilly and I found that Sean stays very cold all the time now) while I maneuvered and adjusted around awkwardly. I did find that over time, putting the non-skid socks on wet feet was much easier for me. I originally thought Sean would be getting dressed in the bedroom, but he preferred the bathroom so he could use his wheelchair for balance and sitting in between every movement. Trial and error.

The bedside commode that we brought home from the hospital was also set up in the bathroom where I thought would be the best location based on how Sean would enter the bathroom. Next to the commode, Kathy moved items from the Amazon boxes and filled a bin with lavender scented toilet bowl liners, sanitary and wet wipes, and briefs. A box of medical gloves sat on the bathroom shelves nearby. You never know when gloves would come in handy. The bin of items next to the bedside commode were all very useful and a good purchase. Having them all nearby and in arms length was also helpful. But as you may have guessed by now, after the first attempt to get him to the bathroom, the commode and bin were being rearranged.

I, once again, didn't consider the amount of room the wheelchair would take up in the bathroom. So, the original spot of being sat up near the actual toilet, now had to be moved smack dab in the middle of the entire bathroom. All of the decorative mats that spruced up the aesthetic of our bathroom had to also be rolled up and moved out so that the wheelchair and Sean wouldn't trip over it. Trial and error.

In the bedroom, Karen unloaded another box and filled a drawer with bed pads and extra grippy-bottomed socks, along with his foot and arm braces that were sent home with him from the hospital and expected to sleep in at night. Tools to help put a shoe on and take a shirt off laid on the dresser and a urinal laid on his nightstand. I wasn't going to take a chance of not making it to the bathroom in the middle of the night because of the time it would take me to get him in there so that was a must to keep nearby. The last box we opened was a gift sent to Sean by my sister, Kimberly. An automatic blood pressure cuff. A gift that I only wish we would have had prior to January 2025. I immediately tested it out on Sean and placed it on a small table right next to him. This gift would be getting a lot of use. Everything had its place and I was proud that I had it all in order.

We finished up with everything that could be done in the moment and Kathy and Ricky headed out.

I finally sat down on the couch and Mike and Karen looked at me and said, "Well, we're headed out, too, and going home for the weekend." My heart stopped and I began to panic. I had no idea that was their plan. They were going to leave me to do this on my own? On the first night? Both boys were with me, but still. I'm sure they noticed my eyes bugging out of my head.

"We just figured you'd like to have the weekend with just the four of you." The thought of just the four of us did sound nice and was the first time it had been that way since Christmas break, but I was still scared if I could really do this on my own. Nothing like being thrown to the wolves. They said their goodbyes and good-lucks and were on their way back to Columbia, Kentucky.

The next big feat I was faced with was bedtime. Similar to the shower, it was trial and error over several weeks, not just that first night. It was a struggle for sure. Similar to putting a baby to bed except this human was almost six feet tall and 190 pounds. Getting him out of the wheelchair and into the bed was challenge number one. It was anything but smooth. His torso fell to the bed, with me directly following and landing on top of him. His legs still dangling off the side of the bed and his right arm laying limp to his side. *Well, I didn't drop him.*

If anything, it gave us a good laugh. So hard in fact that the boys came running into the bedroom to see what was so funny. He was able to help get the left leg up but the right leg was dead weight so I used all my might to lift it up into the bed. The waterproof bed pad that I had positioned in place was now wadded up to the top of the bed. I shimmied the pad back into place while Sean shimmied his body towards the middle of the bed. It was a team effort for sure. Ankle brace on. Arm brace on. Clothes changed. I removed his glasses, pulled the blankets up to his chin, tucked him in and kissed him goodnight. I told him I loved him and he mumbled it back the best that he could.

He was out within 30 minutes. I fell asleep shortly afterwards while laying on my right side looking towards Sean. I no longer had to stare at the box of tissues. Just a month before, I wasn't sure I'd ever see Sean's body laying next to me in our bed again. But there he was and here we were. It was different and it was going to be from here on out and I was coming to that realization. But in that moment as I drifted off, I remember thinking just how thankful I was that even though this was a different version of Sean, he was here with me.

We survived the first day.

———

We'd wake up the next morning to do it all over again. We'd continue to do more trial and error in everything that we'd attempt. The everyday, mundane things that you usually do on autopilot without having to put in any thought, were being relearned. If one way didn't work, no matter how much planning went into it ahead a time, we'd just try again. We'd tweak, adjust, modify or change things as we went along until we found what worked best for us.

And what works best for us may not work the best for you. You can get all the training ahead of time from the therapists, make all the lists, prepare, plan and set things up. But you learn to be okay with it when things don't work out how you thought they would. It will be a lesson you'll learn pretty quickly too. Patience was key during this whole process. That's what trial and error is really. Having the patience to do things many times until you find a successful way to get it done.

Patience taught me adaptation. I learned very quickly after getting home that I was going to have to learn to adapt. Adaptation led to flexibility. Although I've always considered myself a patient person, I definitely had to teach myself to be more flexible. All the things I thought were going to happen and how they were going to happen very rarely worked out that way. No matter how much planning ahead I did. A stroke is anything but planned and that continues to be the case post stroke.

Sean's stroke wanted no part of any organizational and planning skills that I possessed. I've said many times that through Sean's stroke, God is testing all of the weaknesses of my personality, things that before now, I thought were strengths. But I had to learn to take things day by day and sometimes even hour by hour or minute to minute. It is very much a "go with the flow" lifestyle, whether you want it to be that way or not. You have to learn to bend, move and change directions at the last minute to figure things out.

What I thought was going to work perfectly would usually be the things that blow up in my face. This life was going to be full of future trials and errors, because no matter how much I wanted to have control over the situation we were all in, I had zero control. And I was just going to have to be okay with that. The sooner you learn to be okay with it, you'll be miles ahead of where I was during this time. Takeaways: find patience, learn to adapt, be flexible, continue to love and be okay with lots of trial and error.

CHAPTER 11
LEARNING TO CARRY US BOTH

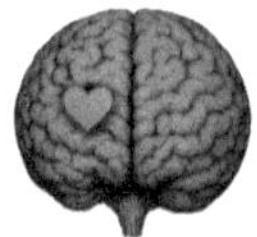

Caregiver. It was the role that I never asked for. The single word that would now be my title and describe exactly who I was. It took precedence over my previous titles of friend, daughter, mom and wife. But it's who I was now and I had to learn to not only power forward in my new role, but to also embrace it, which I did without hesitation and zero questions asked. That old sense of myself no longer matches up to how I will be spending my days moving forward. The person you care for is no longer simply your spouse but also a patient. The disconnect can be disorienting and eye-opening.

I was given the choice to move Sean into a Residential Care Facility versus coming home, but that was never even an option in my mind. He was going to return to his home with his family. That meant more work was going to fall on me and I knew that, but as his wife, I knew it's what I had to do. It's what I wanted to do.

A study conducted by AARP and National Alliance of Caregiving reported that 53 million American adults provide unpaid care to a family member or friend. That is one in every five people. Of those individuals, 22% split their time between full time work and caregiving duties. That would be me. And nearly a quarter of caregivers of a sick adult also have young children under the age of 18. These caregivers belong to the "sandwich generation." Me again. Caregiving duties range from helping with all Activities of Daily Living (ADLs) which is around 96% and 46% performing medical and nursing tasks. Although the number is hard to quantify, a substantial number of caregivers find themselves in this role suddenly and without much lead time or prior planning. Me once again. The numbers are truly astonishing and I am clearly not alone when it comes to taking on the caregiver title and the duties that come along with it. But when you think about it, it makes sense. I'm sure we all know someone who either has cared for someone in the past or is currently doing so. I know I did before I became one myself. But I had no idea how difficult the job would be. Both physically and even more so, mentally. It definitely takes a toll on your body and emotions.

I always assumed that one day I would be a caregiver, but it's natural to assume that that person would probably be an elderly parent. Sean and I had even talked about it and always said we'd avoid sending our parents to an assisted facility if at all possible and would make our home their home. It's what makes the most sense. What doesn't make sense is caregiving for an adult child or your spouse, at least not when you're still in your 40s and are potentially only half way through your life. That is not something that you do plan for. I know it never even crossed my mind. But here I am thrown into it with very little notice. That is the unfortunate side of being a caregiver to someone who has suffered from a stroke, traumatic brain injury and similar injuries.

The only time for planning or training is the period of time they are still in the hospital. I didn't even have a chance to accept the situation before getting the Caregiver title. We do have the hope though that our patient can potentially get better over time. On the flip side, my heart breaks for those caregiving for a family member with cancer, dementia or Alzheimer's, among other similar diseases. A lot of times they are slow oncoming and gradually get worse, being drawn out for decades sometimes. Those caregivers have time to accept their role, get the training and move through the process with time.

Don't get me wrong, being a caregiver sucks no matter how and when you obtained the role. No one is getting a prize for who has it worst. It's not great for anyone, yet so many Americans will take on this role at some point in their lives. It's devastating to me that not only are there so many people that will have to care for someone while watching them suffer and struggle, but that they will go through the trials of neglecting themselves too. The person you are taking care of takes priority, then young children, then maybe your parents, then yourself. The American Cancer Society says that not taking care of yourself as the caregiver is the number one reason for "Caregiver Burnout," which in turn causes you to neglect your own mental and physical health.

I think the fact that I was going to be a caregiver hit me during the last week at Frazier Rehabilitation during Sean's inpatient stay. I was denied my request to get him to stay longer and they were holding firm to the original discharge date. The nurse's aid came in to do their hourly duties of adjusting Sean in the bed, giving him a sponge bath, cleaning him up or just attending to his needs. They were things that I would usually step out of the room for while they took care of him. But stepping out of the room meant that I really didn't know exactly what and how they were doing these things.

I originally would step out to give them privacy (even though our relationship was an open-door policy so to speak) or to spare us both the embarrassment of the situation that he couldn't control and yet another dose of the reality we were in. But with less than a week before going home, I had to know how to do everything. There would be no nurses or aids that I could call on to come in and take care of it for me once we got home.

I walked up to Sean who was laying in the hospital bed and looked him straight in the eyes. He glared back at me so I knew I had his attention. "Look, I know this isn't an ideal situation but it's where we are. In four days, you're coming home and I have to know how to properly take care of you. I'm staying in the room while Tracy cleans you up and I'm going to help her. It's time to rip the bandaid off. We're powering through and we're going to do it together!" I gave him a kiss on the forehead from his wife and put on my caregiver hat.

As much as neither of us wanted to be here, the fact was, we were. So he couldn't argue with my "Come to Jesus" speech. It was what it was.

I proceeded over the last few days at Frazier going from "directional how-tos" to "I'm doing this by myself." The nurse call button was no longer up for grabs to hit. We fought through any embarrassment and the occasional tears and was as ready as I could be to take on caregiving on my own.

My first duty as caregiver after getting things put away at home, was stifling through his medications. Sixteen to be exact. I dumped the two full bags of prescription bottles out on the countertop and began organizing them according to morning, noon and night medications. Karen purchased a large pill box that was fresh out of the packaging and ready to be filled. I spent forty five minutes meticulously sorting through them all and filling up each compartment in the pill box. There were so many, it was easy to make a mistake or just forget where you left off. Off to the side was a stack of nicotine patches. Sean used tobacco from the age of fifteen and began having withdrawals while in the ICU so the patches were added to his daily medication regimen. He had been doing great, and still had a few weeks left weaning down the nicotine dosage before he'd be off for good.

Silver lining about a stroke: it'll scare the shit out of you and (hopefully) break you of any bad habits.

I learned very early on that being a caregiver meant that your needs come very last. I didn't realize that Sean wasn't the only one that lost his independence. I did too and that was a hard thing to accept. It was like moving back in time to when I was caring for a newborn or toddler all over again. It pains me to compare my husband to a child, but there were so many similarities, especially early on. He couldn't be left alone so I was either stuck at home, or I'd have to arrange for someone to be with him. He was learning how to walk, talk, take care of himself and become independent all over again.

His brain had been damaged so that wasn't functioning at full capacity either. That meant, unless he was at therapy, it was me taking on the walking, talking and how-to lessons. I was cleaning up spills, helping him dress, giving him showers, going to the bathroom, all while taking on all the cooking, laundry, running Austin to everywhere he needed to be and going back to work full time.

My "off day" which was on Tuesdays, was far from an off day. It was spent going to doctors appointments, going through medical bills, making phone calls and meetings with attorneys, doctors and case managers. I'd find myself easily spinning in circles and trying to hold it together. I would look forward to going to work honestly. It felt like a break and also where I felt most like myself. It gave me a little bit of normalcy in my now, very chaotic life.

Patience is a virtue as a caregiver. The ability to wait calmly and without getting upset, especially when faced with delays or challenges, is a valuable and admirable quality. And it is definitely a top quality that you must possess or learn to possess as a caregiver. As tired and exhausted as I felt, I honestly was surprised at myself at the amount of patience that I managed to keep. As a matter of fact, it was way more patience than I had with Sean pre-stroke. I think, for me, I saw how much Sean would get frustrated when he couldn't do or say things he could before. Simple things. So, my patience could help cancel out a lot of his frustration. And if by chance, it couldn't, it usually meant the frustration would turn to tears. But I really tried to keep that from happening. That's not to say that my patience wasn't still tested along the way.

I'd finally be able to sit down and he'd have to go to the bathroom which, at the beginning, needed my full assistance. And it wasn't a three minute task, but more like fifteen minutes. Transferring him to the wheelchair (that process alone included lining up the wheelchair to his lounge chair, maneuvering both of us properly, blocking the knee, holding on to his waistband, counting 1-2-3, blocking the right knee, lifting with my legs, getting him in the wheelchair), getting to the commode in the bathroom, doing transfer process all over again, standing him up to pull down the pants, sit him back down, walk out so he could do his business, stand him back up to pull pants back up, sit him back down, transfer process back to his wheelchair, and then transfer process back to the lounge chair. Every single task took ten times as long and required ten times the amount of energy and patience. So, rest time for me is when my head hit the pillow at night, assuming he wouldn't have to go to the bathroom in the middle of the night and do that whole process with my eyes half closed.

A positive of being a caregiver, is you get to witness first hand how your love and care can be motivating to that person. I found I became a cheerleader for Sean. His number one cheerleader in fact. If he expressed his want to try and walk with a cane, I dropped everything to line up chairs in the kitchen, give him a pep talk and let him fly. If he was unsuccessful, we'd try again the next day, but if he was successful, man did we celebrate! Cheering, dancing, hugging and crying tears of joy! They were big moments that I could have missed had I not been there caring for him. Being able to encourage him and cheer him on has been the absolute best and I'm honored to have a front row seat in his recovery. It's times like these that make the exhaustion and heartache all worthwhile.

The good news is that, for Sean and I, what started out as very difficult tasks, got easier over time. And that was with everything bathroom, showers, bedtime, walking, talking. As he grew stronger and his brain began to heal, the tasks became a little easier. That and practice makes perfect, which we did a lot of. I was really leaning into my role as caregiver and was doing a pretty good job at it for the most part. At the same time, I was getting lost in that role and forgetting the role I had before as his wife. I knew and understood my purpose, but was losing myself at the same time. I've researched and read articles and talked to others saying how easy it is, when caregiving for a spouse, to forget that you are also a wife. You are so caught up in the everyday caregiving to make sure they are taken care of and kept safe, that being an actual wife isn't much of a thought.

After several weeks of being home, the wife thought hit me out of nowhere. We were in the shower for the millionth time and I was helping with bathing him. We perfected our routine by that point so we were going through the motions that had become second nature. It hit me while we were in there that Sean hadn't tried coming on to me at all, after all these showers we had been taking together.

Pre-stroke Sean had been banned from the bathroom by me while I was taking a shower because I had absolutely no peace. He'd make flirtatious innuendos, gawking and make suggestive comments, including jumping in the shower with me. After 20 plus years of marriage, I was annoyed by the lack of privacy, but he said I should take it as a compliment that he still found me so attractive. That's a man for you! Gabbing with my homegirls, we'd joke and I'd make the comment about how I could go a year without having sex. How nice it would be to go to bed, and actually just go to bed! Well, that thing that hit me in the shower on that day with Sean? It was Karma. You know nothing good comes from karma. We finished the shower like usual, got dressed and went to bed. I picked up my phone and consulted with my friend, Google.

I avoided looking anything up after Sean's stroke. What I didn't know wouldn't hurt me. But as I laid there in bed in the dark with the Google search bar staring at me, I realized that not a single doctor or nurse ever mentioned anything to me (or Sean) about intimacy after a stroke. How strange. It is a natural part of life and very important within a marriage or relationship. Had we not shown them by our actions, that we were in a happy and loving marriage? Is that why nothing was ever said to us? To be fair, up until that day, it had never even crossed my mind. My mind was just on saving Sean and keeping him alive, not if we could ever have sex again. But as he was getting better, I did start thinking about it. We were only in our 40s for goodness sakes, still young and very much in love.

"Intimacy after a stroke," I hesitantly typed the words in the search bar. And just as I suspected and why I hadn't talked to my Google friend before, I was not thrilled with the results. It mentioned that intimacy can look different after a stroke, including hand holding and cuddling. *What!?* That's not what I wanted to see. Discouraged, I turned off my phone and sat it on my nightstand, vowing to myself to never search the subject again. Over the next month, I kept that vow I made and showers continued as normal. The new normal, that is. Some of my girlfriends finally were brave enough to ask me the question regarding sex. "Absolutely nothing." I'd solemnly respond and they, too, looked bummed for me. Damn you karma!

It was late April. It had been an overall really good day for Sean. That was the day he asked to try and walk for the first time. And he did it! Then he wanted to walk without my help. And he did it! I recorded him to send to all the family so everyone could celebrate with him! He said it was the first time he felt weight on his right leg. You could see through the tears, the hope in his eyes. He was seeing the progress himself and he needed that boost of confidence. And that confidence carried right into that night's shower.

He sat on his shower bench and I proceeded to wash my own hair, paying no attention to him really.

When I rinsed the suds out of my hair and washed the soap off my face, I opened my eyes. Sean was looking at me with his pre-stroke eyes, not his post-stroke ones. That flirtatious crooked grin popped on his face. A grin I had seen thousands of times before. In that moment, I was able to step out of being his caregiver. I got to just be Sean's wife. Something we had both desperately missed and needed. Something that was going to keep us moving forward.

CHAPTER 12

LOVE AND GRACE

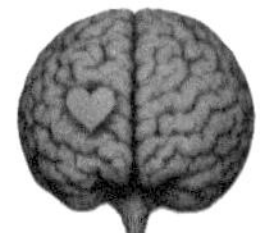

"Make sure you take care of yourself." I was maybe 24 hours into Sean's stroke when someone said this to me for the first time. My initial reaction was to do a full on eye roll. *Myself?* I didn't even know who that was and that early on I was only thinking about Sean. As the days, weeks and months went on, I would hear that statement more and more. And I absolutely hated that sentence. Like, hated it. I began to even start resenting my friends and family that would say it to me. I know they were only looking out for me and were concerned about my well being, but taking care of myself was the last thing on my mind.

I knew better though, especially working in the industry of self care. Lord knows, I've said that same statement to countless people and guests that would see me for massages while taking care of a loved one. I had no idea how annoying I probably sounded to them. I found out real quick that giving that piece of advice was much easier than receiving it. Even though I would cringe when someone would tell me that, I knew they were right. But it didn't make it any less irritating.

I remember thinking at one point when I was told to take care of myself for the one millionth time, Sean had only been home for a few weeks. He was still needing 24/7 assistance with literally everything. Did I want a break? YES! Did I want to go somewhere else besides work and doctor's appointments? YES! Did I want just a moment of time to myself? YES! But it wasn't as simple as taking off to go do the things that I knew I so desperately wanted and needed. I mean, I had offers from friends to come hang out with Sean so I could go out, which was generous. But when I'd get those offers that truly came from a place of love, all I could think about was the lists of things that would be required of them to just "sit with Sean." It was so much more than that. They don't know how to safely transfer him. And what if he needs to go to the bathroom? Are they going to be willing to take on the responsibilities of what is required for that? Doubt it. And Sean definitely wouldn't feel comfortable with it. So I was kind of stuck between a place I wanted to run from and a place where I wanted to be.

I want to back-up to Sean's time in the ICU. When I first came to the realization that I did need to find a way to take care of myself was that moment that I found myself in the dimly lit hospital stairwell hysterically crying. You could hear nothing but the echoes of medical staff's heavy footsteps from several floors down and my crying.

Kelly was there with me that day and when I emerged from the stairway door, she looked at me and said, "Have you started your therapy yet?" I had been so concerned about Sean, that I did forget about myself, which is so easy to do in situations like this. But I knew if I continued to go down this path without an outlet of my own, I would spiral out of control quickly. I promised Kelly that I would make an appointment and she held me accountable. She didn't leave me that day until I made the call to my therapist. I was able to miraculously get in with her for a phone call the very next day.

I sat on the shower bench in Sean's private bathroom attached to his room at Frazier and cried through my entire therapy call. He was in physical therapy learning to move again and I was in mental therapy learning to cope with life again. The familiar sound of the echoing tears rang out once again, and it was decided at that time that regular bi-weekly calls with her were non-negotiable. I was too exhausted to argue so I put up no fight and found myself looking forward to the next call before I even hung up with that one. The release I got during that one hour call was so freeing.

I already had several doctor's appointments for myself scheduled out during the first month that Sean got home. These were all scheduled before Sean's stroke occurred. It would have been super easy for me to cancel those appointments. After all, I didn't really have the time. My time was already spread super thin taking care of Sean and all of the business side of things that come up when medical tragedy strikes. But I kept those appointments anyway. I was no good taking care of Sean if, God forbid, something was wrong with me. So I got the mammogram, the dermatologist check, the lab work, the dentist, the pap smear and the neurological check. I was diagnosed with epilepsy in 2002 and had been seizure-free since then, but would also be more likely to get them if under high amounts of stress. I was cleared from any issues, but when I started crying to my gynecologist in the middle of my exam – yes, that's right, crying while my feet were in stirrups and the scratchy paper gown gaped open across my chest. She strongly encouraged me to talk to my primary care physician.

Within a few days, I was put on a mild antidepressant and anxiety medications. I was never one to turn to prescription drugs during the tough times of life, but I definitely needed a little help to get me through this time. And that's okay. I really didn't have anything to be ashamed of. I was adamant that Sean be put on an antidepressant when he started struggling mentally, so I needed to take my own advice. And I'm giving the same advice if you find yourself in a similar situation. At the very least, let your self care be simply getting a doctor check-up. It will help keep you sane and hopefully take care of anything before they become issues. The last thing your sick loved one needs is for you to be laying in the bed next to them.

Early on, my Homegirls had to force me to do things for myself. It helped that we had been friends for such a long time because they didn't care if I told them no, which I did. They were either going to take me anyway or just show up at my door. One week into Sean's ICU stay, it was Landon's night to stay with Sean. I was tired and just wanted to go home and cry myself to sleep. I definitely didn't feel like doing any sort of celebrating. At that time, anything outside of being at the hospital or sleeping felt like celebrating. I wouldn't even allow myself to listen to music in the car. Music can bring joy, and I didn't really want to even feel that emotion. But the Homegirls insisted that I needed some "girl time."

They showed up that Friday night at my door with snacks, drinks and their company. Those that couldn't attend were sending pictures or on Facetime. I found myself slowly relaxing and wouldn't you know it, even laughing. The night only lasted a couple of hours but, oh, how I needed that time. I didn't know I needed it, but they did. For that short time, I forgot that my world was falling apart. I was able to escape reality for two whole hours. Don't fight off friends or family that want to help you escape. It's what you want to do, but just allow yourself to give in. I promise you'll be glad you did.

Guilt. Such a strong emotion that rears its ugly head when you actually think about doing something for yourself. As women, I think that's an emotion that's engrained in most of us early on. We might go through a selfish phase, but for the most part we tend to put ourselves second, third or even last. Children, your job, spouse and parents all seem to come before me, myself and I. And why is that?

Men don't seem to have that problem. I haven't experienced many instances when a man feels really bad for leaving to go play golf, or a child feels bad for asking to get something for themselves at the store when they're out shopping for others or a boss asks you to cancel your personal plans in order to stay and do something for them. Women are statistically more likely to be primary caregivers, so it's no big surprise when we are actually in that role and when we want to do something for ourselves, Guilt takes over.

I mentioned earlier not to fight off those trying to encourage you to have self care time. But you do have permission to fight the Guilt. It may knock you down several times, give you a black eye or a bloody lip, but keep getting back up. You can compromise with Guilt, but don't let it win. Right at the six-month anniversary of Sean's stroke, Kasey had an extra room in her vacation condo in Florida and she asked me to come down for a couple of days. I so desperately needed the break. I began fantasizing about sitting on the porch of the Floridian home, looking at the ocean and listening to the waves while holding a cup of coffee. And then looking at the same scenery with a glass of wine during sunset. But the evil Guilt emotion overtook the mere thought of surf and sand.

I talked to my therapist about it, and began to cry. I honestly didn't realize that the guilty feeling had even grabbed on to me so tightly until I started to talk about it out loud. Even though I wanted the short vacation, the last thing I wanted was for Sean to think I was trying to get away from him because he was a burden. Or that I didn't want to take him with me because he was a burden. I would have been absolutely crushed if my fear were true. My therapist encouraged me to mention it to Sean and talk it over with him.

Later that day while casually bobbing around in the pool, I said to him, "Kasey invited me to come down to Florida with her for a few days. Your parents would stay with you while I was gone. What do you think?" Without a single moment of hesitation, do you know what he said?

"I'd be pissed." Even with his aphasia, I understood exactly what he said.

Well, that sealed the deal right there. Guilt held on tightly and refused to let go. In fact, it was strangling me. Before the stroke, I did frequent girls trips and he never once had an issue with it. Time away from one another was always prioritized almost as much as time together, as long as we could afford it. We encouraged one another to do things with just our friends. He needed me now, though, and even if his parents were perfectly capable of staying with him, the guilt still wouldn't allow me to go. So, as much as I'd like to tell you I hopped on a flight to Florida, I did not. But I still refused to let Guilt win.

As the months passed, I started giving myself permission to do a little more self care. Sometimes, it was a walk around the neighborhood or meeting a girlfriend after work for an "emergency cocktail hour," or scheduling a pedicure when I knew Landon would be home. That also meant not just giving massages at work, but getting back into the habit of receiving massages. As a massage therapist, I know the benefits go far beyond working out knots and kinks in the actual muscles. It works out the emotional and mental kinks too.

I travel about 45 minutes to Bardstown, Kentucky to get my massages. Bardstown is a cute town known as the "Bourbon Capital of the World" filled with friendly southerners, clothing boutiques, quaint coffee houses and ice cream shops. I balled up my fist and took a hard swing at *guilt*. I pulled up my friend Google, and searched for local hotels in Bardstown. I found a boutique hotel just minutes away from the spa I went to. Before Guilt picked himself back up, I hit "book now" and entered in my credit card number. Guilt's best friend, Regret, immediately showed up to the fight. Regret knew that doing something like this was way out of my comfort zone, but I knew I needed to do this for myself, and in turn for Sean. It was going to make me a better person, caregiver and wife.

Four days before the six month stroke-aversary, I got my much-needed and well-deserved massage. Afterwards, I drove myself to downtown Bardstown and walked around the town square, grabbing an iced coffee and a box of homemade macaroons that tasted like small droplets from heaven in my mouth. I savored each sip and each bite of the sweetness. I visited the little stores and talked to the locals. I went to the library and wrote out a chapter of this book you are reading now. I checked into the hotel and laid by the pool. I got dinner that night at the restaurant on the property and brought it back to my room. I gave myself a facial and a pedicure and watched a chick flick movie. I turned my alarm off and woke up the next morning when my body said it was time.

For twenty four hours, I focused solely on myself. I pushed Guilt and Regret aside and only left room for Love to come in. Love for myself. Love for the woman that was being put last because everyone else needed her a little more. Strokes are no fun and can suck the life out of you, but don't let it take your love. You can't pour love from an empty cup. Self care is not an indulgence, it's a necessity. Fill your own cup with love first, so that you have love to give to others. Win the fight.

Just like the best friend relationship between Guilt and Regret, Love's best friend is Grace. Yes, I'm not only telling you to love yourself, but to also give yourself Grace. For me personally, giving myself Grace is harder than giving myself Love. By now, you should have a good idea of my personality and who I am as a person, so it shouldn't come as a surprise when I tell you that it is very hard for me to give myself Grace. I'm a perfectionist and like to be in control; control of others, myself and situations. But strokes hold all the control and leave hardly anything left over. So when I had to learn to "go with the flow," that also meant finding

Grace to give myself. When things didn't go the way I wanted, or Sean didn't like how I did things, I would give myself a lot of grief.

There would be many times when I felt like a failure. I felt like a failure when I couldn't transfer Sean without stumbling, or if I couldn't understand him when he so badly wanted to tell me something. When I had to take back the cooking duties (that had become one of Sean's passions), I overcooked the pork chops. They were chewy and tough, and admittedly pretty bad. Add it to the failure list. When I appealed a medical bill and it was denied, I felt like a failure. I was failing Sean and failing myself. It was a horrible feeling. I'd talk to my friends about it, listen to a podcast on the subject or bring it up in my therapy sessions. The common theme they all told me was "give yourself Grace."

I learned I wasn't necessarily failing, even though at the time, it's what it felt like. I had to remind myself that I was taking on a lot. When you're in the day to day, you tend to forget everything on your plate when tragedy strikes your family. I was simply doing what I needed to do for everyone to survive. I was working full time, being the primary caregiver to Sean, primary chauffeur to Austin's busy teenage life and handling all the household duties and finances. In addition to that, I was learning to take on what used to be Sean's responsibilities; home repairs, car maintenance, watering the flowers and pool maintenance. What should have been a simple battery change in our home security system, ended up anything but easy. The alarm squealed the high pitch tone, I couldn't get it turned off and apparently didn't hear my phone ring when the security company called. Next thing I know, a fire truck and fireman were at my front door. At least Sean found the whole ordeal amusing.

I was also taking on all of the new responsibilities that came with a disabled spouse who was in the hospital for over a month. I often thought of that scene in the movie "Bruce Almighty" starring Jim Carrey. If you haven't seen it, I'll paint you a picture. In response to a strain of bad luck and blaming God for his shortcomings, Jim Carrey's character Bruce, accepts the challenge of taking over God's job for a week to see if he can do any better. He first uses his newfound Godly powers for selfish gain, getting designer clothes and fancy cars and impressing his girlfriend with lavish dates. Bruce soon realizes that having God's power is more complex than he imagines. He struggles to answer all the prayers, or in my case all the demands and responsibilities that lie solely on my shoulders to take care of.

Bruce attempts to find ways to organize the prayers. First, he "commands" them to a file cabinet. When he opens the file, the drawer knocks him over with such force and cabinets continue to fill the room. He then "commands" the prayers to be in the form of post-it notes, but they fill an entire room with no open space available, blowing away in the wind. Finally, he "commands" them to email, which seems like a good idea. All of the prayers are now neatly organized on a computer. He downloads the prayers. Over 1.5 million pop up. He proceeds to answer the prayer emails with lightning, Godly speed. Pressing the "Enter" button and looking as if he completed his task, he's met with an updated list of 3.5 million new prayers.

I can't tell you the amount of times I felt like Bruce. I'd complete three things, only to go to the mailbox to five envelopes waiting for me to take care of. I'd pay off some medical bills only to receive a stack of letters from a collections agency for the few I hadn't paid. I received a letter with the good news that Sean got a spot for a Brain Waiver program only to be told I had to jump through the hundreds of hoops that are Medicaid requirements. Terminating a relationship with one attorney only to have to possibly get another one. I just couldn't stay afloat and the feeling of drowning was taking over causing me not to be able to breathe. I needed saving by Grace.

Once I did find it and allowed it in next to Love, I was able to tackle my plate of responsibilities better. It allowed me not to get worked up and anxious so easily. Now I won't say that finding Grace allowed for all those things to disappear. They never left if I'm being honest, but they're also not as prominent as they were in the beginning. Grace has moved them from the forefront to the background and I'm able to take on everything a little easier. Because I am only one person and I choose to give myself Grace.

Find the old you in the new you. The Caregiver you. Kat McGowan, a journalist who focuses on caregiving and has also been a caregiver for multiple family members, wrote an article about how Caregiving can test you, body and soul. She made a profound statement that I wholeheartedly agree with and continue to give myself the same advice. It only makes sense that I pass on her wisdom on the subject.

She states, "Given the emotional weight of the role, caregivers are often told to practice self-care. Caregiver identity theory suggests another approach: Think about who you were before, who you are now, and how those two yous relate. Because, if the existential pain of caregiving is due to a gap between who you think you're supposed to be (your old self), and who you are now (caregiver self), you need to bridge the gap."

How are you going to bridge the gap? If you find yourself in a similar position where you have fallen upon a situation that piles on the stress and pressure alongside the guilt and regret, stop and take a moment.

- Give yourself a pep talk. Positive affirmations can go a long way.
- Buy yourself the fancy coffee or a special treat at your local bakery. Lord knows, you deserve it!
- Call a friend to talk on the phone while walking the dog.
- Schedule a therapy appointment.

- Take a bath. Not just a bath to get clean, but a *therapeutic* bath. Light a candle, turn off the lights and play some soothing music.
- Do a short devotion and spend time with God.
- Simply take five extra minutes in the morning to just breathe. Like, actually let the only sound that you hear be the inhale and exhale of your own breath. A good rule of thumb is to inhale through the nose for four seconds, hold your breath for seven seconds, and exhale slowly out of your mouth for eight seconds.
- Give yourself grace and self love. No matter how hard it is, make the time. Find the time. It's there, but you have to fight to find it sometimes because it is buried deep down under Guilt and Regret and the others. You may not be able to take twenty four hours, but make a little time for yourself. It's a long road ahead and if your cup is filled with the good stuff, there won't be any room for the things to take you down.

"I hope you are learning to give yourself the credit you deserve. I hope you are beginning to recognize just how strong you are for pulling yourself through each and every difficult time in your life. I hope you allow this realization to walk with you, alongside any obstacles or roadblocks you might encounter along your journey. I hope you know just how much you are capable of and that no matter how challenging a situation may seem, you have the courage to keep moving, to keep growing, and to keep healing. I hope you realize just how incredible you are, and just how much you deserve your own love."

— Charlotte Freeman

CHAPTER 13

ACCEPTING THE HELP

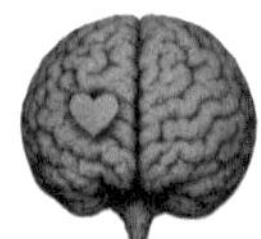

I sat at a small table in U of L Hospital's cafeteria. Kathy and Austin sat across from me and Kelly sat to the right of me. We were on day three of being in the ICU and they were forcing me to get out of the room and get something to eat. I was in a complete fog and daze, barely present in the conversation at the cafe's table.

Kelly spoke up, "I want to talk to you about money. A lot of people want to help you and Sean and the family." I sat still looking straight ahead instead of at her. "The girls and I have been coming up with ways to assist you all during this time so you can spend time with Sean and it can be one less thing for you to worry about."

I made eye contact with Kathy. She knew exactly what I was thinking, but I could tell she was begging me to listen to Kelly.

I mumbled, "No, I can't ask people to give me money." Just the thought of it made my skin crawl. We were never ones to ask for handouts, and were proud we worked hard for what we had. But I'd be lying if I said that the thought of paying all the bills that were still going to continue to come in made my stomach twist into knots. I would figure it out though. I always seemed to.

"Erin, please let us help you," Kelly was more making a statement versus asking. I knew that all the homegirls had a separate group text that I wasn't a part of where they pulled in Laura, Ricky, Ali and others to concoct up several small plans into one large master plan. By the time it got back to me, the decision was already made or the deed had already been done. I was simply being told about it at that point. Our friends came together to make sure it was one less thing I had to worry about or make a decision on. And they also probably knew that if they truly asked me, I'd respond with "No." The last thing I wanted to do was put anyone out of their way or inconvenience them.

Kelly continued, telling me about all the small plans they had been working on. She spoke with such care and empathy, but it was so much. I literally was unable to comprehend all of the information she was giving me. My body turned hot, I was feeling over-whelmed and everything was going numb. It was all building up until I broke down sobbing right at the lunch table. I just couldn't take it all in and I felt so extremely guilty for the ideas that she was just suggesting me to take advantage of. All of the help that she wanted me to just accept with no questions asked.

Then she capped it off with, "You would do this for us so let us do this for you." Well, I couldn't argue with that. Our friends were like extended family and we would do anything for them.

Still crying, I gave up and gave in to her requests. "Okay." I still couldn't make myself ask for the help though, especially with the financial side of things, but it was completely pointless to continue arguing with Kelly. Plus, I didn't have the energy.

Anyone that knows me, knows that I worry easily and Lord knows, I had an endless list of worries on my plate. Although I had gotten better about worrying over anything and everything the last few years, Sean's stroke brought in a hurricane of worries that were hitting me in the face, and I couldn't avoid them no matter how hard I tried. So maybe it wasn't such a bad idea to let our friends take some of those on for me.

My boss, Laura, organized a Valentine's fundraiser event at the salon to provide mini pampering services where the proceeds would go to us. All of the staff came in on their days off to provide these services to our guests. They donated their time so that others could donate financially. Afterwards, Laura presented me with an envelope of cash and a stack of cards filled with food delivery, grocery and gas gift cards. The cards were filled with heartfelt notes and prayers. I would stay up late in the hospital room after Sean fell asleep and read each and every one of them. I kept all the cards and taped them to the wall by his bed to greet him when he returned home. I wanted him to see all the support, love and encouragement he was getting, because after all, he had no idea what all was being done for us while he laid helpless in the hospital bed.

The Homegirls worked together to set up pay accounts for people to donate funds to help us out. I was brought to tears many times by the generosity of others and it will never be forgotten. These weren't just people that were in our lives presently. They were high school friends, people from a church I was once a member of, old co-workers, ex bosses, acquaintances and the most shocking, complete strangers. Sean's stroke touched so many people and they all just wanted to help. They wanted to help us because Sean is such an amazing person, friend, son, dad and husband. And that was evident with all the support we received.

Ricky planned a golf scramble fundraiser for late summer, spending weeks getting sponsors, food and drinks donated so the profits could go to us to help with the home and medical bills flooding in. Another positive with an event like this was that Sean was eight months post stroke and was moving around a little better. He was starting to regain enough strength, both physically and mentally, that he could actually converse with everyone that came to support him and thank them personally. Up until this event, he really didn't get to see first hand the support he had received. I think it gave him a boost of confidence and encouragement to continue to put in the hard work!

Social media can be used for good or for evil. If you're on it, which 73% of Americans are, you already know this. It can be very deceitful and damaging, but can also be helpful. When I made that first post about Sean's stroke, the news spread like wildfire. Good news travels fast, but it seems that bad news travels even faster. I was expected to give an update every night on Sean's condition. If not, I would be blasted with texts or calls, and I simply didn't have the time or energy to respond to everyone, but I wanted to. So, every night after Sean would fall asleep and I laid in either the hard lounger listening to the beeping of the ICU machines or in our bed next to the box of kleenexes, I'd give the Sean update on social media. I would then drift off and wake up to hundreds of comments. Comments with a lot of prayer hands or strong arm emojis or words of encouragement. But I'd also get words of thanks for taking the time to give the update.

Through my updates, I began receiving private messages from people, past and present in our lives, offering ways they could help.

An old massage guest of mine from over ten years ago sent me a message.

> We have a brand new electric wheelchair. We got it for my dad who passed before using it. We would love to give it to Sean to use once he gets home.

They delivered that wheelchair to us two days after Sean arrived home. They refused to take anything for it and were just so happy it was going to someone that could use it. Wow. The gift made me speechless. It was more than just a lavish donation. It gave Sean some independence to move about the house on his own, during a time when 24/7 assistance was required. And when your independence is stripped from you in an instant, any little bit that you can get is a huge deal.

Then I received a message from a past School of Rock parent.

> I wanted to let you know that I reached out to
> Steve, the Stroke Survivor in the Frazier video
> you posted. He wanted me to let you know he'd
> be happy to come visit with you and Sean to talk
> to you all about his experience and offer any
> support he can. I'm happy to connect you.

Hell yeah! I jumped all over that, especially when I received that message when Sean was dealing with his bouts of depression. Within the week, Steve personally came up to Frazier, stood next to Sean's bed and gave one of the best pep talks you can give. After all, Steve was Sean just a few years prior. But here he was walking and talking and working and driving. I needed that visit just as much as Sean did. He was such a positive testament and inspiration that we so desperately needed when it looked like there wasn't an end in sight. And to this day, Steve still checks in on Sean.

Shirley's Way, a local organization, heard about Sean and reached out to me wanting to help too. In a round-about way, I think it was a mutual friend on Facebook that made the connection on our behalf. Shirley's Way is a passionate, community-driven nonprofit committed to raising funds that directly support individuals courageously battling cancer and other disabilities. Their mission is rooted in compassion and focused on anything that improves the well-being of our community. They proudly support families across Kentucky and Southern Indiana. Since 2014, they've given away almost $9 million dollars to the community. The founder, Mike Mulrooney, started Shirley's Way after his mother was diagnosed with liver cancer and made it his personal mission to help others with the financial strain that comes along with cancer and other tragic disabilities. He not only set up a donation page on our behalf, but kicked off the funding with $3,500. He donated t-shirts that the girls designed that could be sold where all the proceeds would go to us as well.

Help doesn't just come in the form of monetary donations. The way to the heart is through food. Even if I was struggling to eat, there was no chance I, nor anyone else in the immediate family, was going hungry. Full meals were being dropped off at the hospital while other people were sneaking in the house to put food in our fridge. And if the fridge was full, frozen lasagnas and casseroles were saved in the freezer to have at a later date. School of Rock, where Austin attended for drum lessons, set up a food train once Sean got home and we had home-cooked meals every few days with plenty of leftovers. We didn't buy or make a single meal for over three months. It was just another thing that everyone wanted to make sure I didn't have to worry about. It was help.

We had people offering to run to the grocery and picking up items we needed, driving Austin to all of his lessons and school activities and things being done around the house. A cleaning company showed up to clean the house several times so I didn't have to worry about when and how the house would get cleaned. Home-girls' husbands were installing ramps and handicap bars and hanging things up. They were things that Mike would have usually done, but he'd be so exhausted too when he got home from his appointments, so all of the "handyman jobs" were helpful to him too.

The only thing I specifically asked for was coffee every morning and Sara made sure I was greeted with my caffeine the moment I woke up, which was the fuel that was really keeping me going. That, and prayers. I mentioned at one point that my eyes were raw from all the crying. The next day, I had an iced down cooler of moisturizing eye gels to put under my eyes. If something was just mentioned in passing that we might need or want, there were sets of ears that were listening, taking notes and making it happen within 24 hours. We literally wanted for nothing. I was glad that I finally gave in and accepted the help. Because once I did, I got to cross off some worries on my list, which you know I love. And I got to see how there are still a lot of wonderful people in this world, and we are just lucky a lot of those people are in our lives.

The gift of time can be a huge help. I know for most there are not enough hours in the day to take care of the long list of items that are on your own list of things to do. Time is precious and valuable, but our parents donated so much of their time after Sean's stroke. Yes, they are retired and our parents but they still have lives. Mike and Karen canceled the month-long trip to Florida that they look forward to every February because they knew I was going to need them. I didn't ask them to cancel their trip, but they did without hesitation, even risking losing $4,000.

Even though Sean is a grown man, he's still their baby and they wanted to be there to care for him when I could not. I know I'll feel that way about Landon and Austin as they grow older. For the first six weeks after Sean's stroke, they only went home for two nights. Otherwise, they were either at the hospital relieving me or back at home, helping around the house. The same goes for Kathy. I think she only missed coming up to the hospital one day. Her time was spent taking on the Sean shifts no one else could and offering a calming presence for me during such a stressful time. She wouldn't necessarily force her way into things, but she made sure she was always there if and when I needed her.

Once Sean came back home in March, I was able to arrange for Mike and Karen to go home more, but they'd come in every

Wednesday in time to pick Sean up from his day of therapy, stay with him all day Thursday and then transport him back and forth to therapy on Fridays. This allowed me to go to work, which was the only thing allowing me to feel normal at that time. Since Sean needed so much assistance early on, the lifting was left to either me or Mike. Karen would pick up around the house or do a load of laundry and Kathy was on call to get Austin to all of his activities or bring over dinner.

Gradually, as Sean continued to get better and stronger, I was slowly able to back them off from such an intense schedule, as he was able to be left alone for short periods of time. But I can't even begin to add up the hours and days of their time that they gave us. There is no amount of money to put on that and it was one of the best gifts I could have asked for. It was help that I happily accepted because I knew I wasn't going to be able to do it alone. I'll never be able to express my gratitude for their gift of time.

Help doesn't have to come in the form of material things. If somebody you love is facing a medical crisis and you have a personality or business strength or a connection of some sort that would be helpful, offer that up. I mentioned in Part One how timing played a big part in Sean's stroke — me finding Sean when I did and Sara still working at U of L. The third case of divine timing that helped us so much was Kelly. Kelly worked as VP of Human Resources with her company for the last five years and always held a position in the HR department before then. She has handled things from training, benefits, hiring, firing, enforcing rules and everything in between. Those are her strengths and she's extremely good at what she does. Due to her company merging with another, her job was eliminated the December prior to Sean's stroke. Her plan was to take a month or two off prior to searching for her next job opportunity. She had no idea that she would become my personal HR representative one month into her job transition period.

In my personal experience, the hospital staff gives you about 48 hours to take everything in about your loved one's condition before they hit you with papers, brochures, pamphlets and applications. That's right. While you've barely started processing everything, you are getting hit in every direction with the business side of things and are expected to make clear, reasonable decisions. Which on a regular basis, I'm perfectly capable of doing. But I was far from capable in that moment. Insert Kelly. She swooped in, once again without even being asked, and helped me during my time of need. She showed up every day to the hospital with her laptop and set up her own little office in the corner of the ICU waiting room. She participated in every conversation that I had with the Stroke unit case manager, asked questions that I didn't even know needed to be asked, took the notes and set up the accounts.

There was one day where I ventured out of the cold ICU room and walked down the hall to stretch my legs. I walked into the waiting room to greet the visitors that were there at the time. I looked over and there was Kelly in her makeshift corner office, typing away and writing on a notepad.

The phone was up to her ear and she said, "Hi, my name is Erin Troklus and I'm calling to inquire about your services. My husband had a stroke and…" There she was chatting away and gathering information for me, not skipping a beat. She was being "HR Kelly." Karen sat in the opposite corner of the waiting room and giggled at her deceitful, but well intentioned tactics. She was in business mode and she wasn't slowing down.

Before she'd leave each day, she'd debrief me on all her findings. "You'll want to proceed with this company. I've set you up an account. Here is your username and password. This company is a waste of time, you don't need them. I've emailed Sean's employer and we'll sit down and call them together tomorrow. They have to do this for him because he is disabled, but we'll also want to inquire about x, y and z. I filled this application out but I just need you to fill out the personal financial information and Sean's social security number." While my head was spinning on the ground, Kelly's was firmly in place and she was getting shit done. Shit that I couldn't even think about doing, but needed to happen. She was saving my time and sanity. She literally took care of everything so I could just be with Sean. That alone was worth accepting her help.

Being the wife, I had to be on the call with Sean's employer the following day. We found a small, private break room on a different unit. Kelly made the call and we put his HR rep on speaker. My body was present at the meeting, but my mind wasn't. Thankfully, my HR rep was present as well. Kelly sat with her notepad ready to take notes and fire off questions if needed. I was so fortunate that she had such extensive Human Resources knowledge because she knew exactly what Sean's employer SHOULD say and what they SHOULD do for him and me. I'm happy to pass on her expertise to you.

If you find yourself in this situation and you are on a call with your loved one's employer and you don't have a Kelly in the meeting with you, here are some questions that you should consider asking. The first question would be if they qualify for the Family Medical Leave Act (FMLA). FMLA provides unpaid job protection for up to three months for certain family and medical reasons, a stroke being one of them. If the employee has worked for the company for over twelve months, they are qualified to receive FMLA and the company is required to offer FMLA by law if they employ over fifty employees and they have worked a minimum of 1250 hours during that first year.

Unfortunately, in Sean's instance, he had only been with his company for four months, so he did not qualify for FMLA. But he was able to apply for accommodations under The Americans with Disabilities Act (ADA). Sean's employer was kind enough to hold his position for three months, to then be reviewed again at that time, but that is not a requirement for employers to do under ADA. If, after the three months, he could have returned to work but with restrictions, the ADA would allow him to, providing reasonable accommodations, if applicable. Any employer that has more than fifteen employees has to abide by ADA regulations. There wouldn't be much of a need to apply for both if they qualify for FMLA, however if they were able to return to work after the three month time frame, it may be beneficial to apply for ADA at that time.

The second question would be to find out if the employer offers any other type of benefits that would be helpful in the situation. Do they offer Short Term Disability (STD) and/or Long Term Disability (LTD)? If so, gather the info on the provider of those plans and start the process immediately. STD policies are usually three or six months long, with LTD kicking in afterwards, assuming that benefit was available. These policies offer a partial payroll protection that can allow for some money to continue coming in while the employee is out of work.

Ask the employer if they have any ancillary benefits such as hospital stay coverage, accident coverage or critical illness coverage? These are usually voluntary benefits that the employee would have had to sign up for and pay a monthly premium on. Unfortunately for Sean, he did not choose to participate in any of these. Therefore, we potentially lost out on thousands of dollars that could have been paid out, often in one lump sum. But just like any other type of insurance, it's a gamble if you choose to participate in any of these plans or not. More than likely, it won't affect you, but it can and will affect some.

Does the employee have Paid Time Off (PTO) still available? Luckily, Sean did have some PTO so I was able to get the appropriate forms filled out and sent back to his employer. This allowed PTO to be used to supplement the remaining amount that STD did not cover to be able to continue getting a full paycheck for a short period of time. Unfortunately, since he was new to the company, he didn't have a lot of PTO built up but he did have some.

When the time comes where the employer can no longer hold the position because the employee's return to work date is still very unknown (which was Sean's case), the company will have to terminate their employment. You'll want to find out at that point how long the health insurance and other benefits last once the termination is finalized. Please note that I would not bring up this question during the initial meeting! You'll know if it's going to come down to that as you see how your loved one is recovering. No sense in planting a bug in their ears about something that you don't even know will happen for sure or not. Take care of the other things now, and worry about this down the road.

Sean's employer finally had to terminate him on June 1st, a little over four months post stroke. Honestly, it was very generous of them to give him that long. His health insurance coverage would end on June 30th. That gave me a month to research other insurance options for myself, the boys and Sean. I chose to keep Sean on a COBRA plan. The up side to COBRA is it continues on with the very same coverage that he had all along (it's just paying a third party to keep that insurance coverage). Seeing as how we met the deductible before the end of January and he continued to have multiple doctor and therapy appointments, it only made sense to keep him on that policy. The downside to COBRA? It's extremely expensive. Like ridiculously expensive. If I wanted to keep all four of us on COBRA, it was going to cost me $2,000 per month. No way I could afford that. I don't know anyone that can afford that! So, I chose to find a separate policy through an insurance agent for myself and the boys that was a little more affordable. Moving on to the worst case scenario. If God forbid, your loved one passes from their illness, many employers offer life insurance so you'd want to inquire about that.

I know that is a lot. And unfortunately, it's just the tip of the iceberg of things that you will have to consider, but I hope this will at least provide you with a "heads up" and guideline on the right questions to ask and the information to gather if you don't have a Kelly in your life that can assist you with these items. She gave me a gift that I'll never be able to repay her for. I'm really not sure I could have survived that time without her and her knowledge. So, I'm paying forward that gift. Let me be your Kelly.

When Sean would have a good day, I would have a good day. And each day, for the most part, would be baby steps better than the day before. That meant that I was able to be a little more focused on all the HR and business items. My head was clearer, I could focus more and make a phone call without Kelly being present. I could take care of the shit that she had been doing for me. My big girl panties were up and on tight by the time she accepted a new job position in March and I was ready to take over where she left off and get things done. And in case you were wondering what her new job was…it was head of a Human Resources department that didn't even exist yet. She was able to create it from the ground up. Perfect job and perfect timing.

Accept the help. I know your instinct may be to say no, it was mine anyways. It was almost a good thing I didn't have the energy to argue with anyone because once I received the help, it was such a relief. And my advice to you if you are the friend of someone going through a tragedy it would be to just do it. If you ask, you'll more than likely be told no.

Don't say, "Let me know if there is anything that you need." I am 99% sure you will not hear back from them, even though there really are things that they need. And don't ask the open ended question of "What do you need help with?" Because the answer is "Everything" but the answer you'll get is nothing. I'd even often respond with, "Your prayers are all we need." And although that was true, there was a literal and mental pile of things stacking up over to the side, staring me down but unseen by most. Instead, pop in and just drop off food — they are hungry and they will eat it. Or show up with a cup of coffee in hand. Or just anticipate their needs. My Homegirls dropped off an overnight bag with every possible thing you can think of — a cardigan, travel toiletries, sanitary wipes, vitamin C gummies, hair clips, Liquid IV water packets, a comfy bra, house slippers, a throw blanket, tissues and of course, my trusty journal with a box of pens. Other friends dropped off puzzle books, quick snacks or a deck of cards. Every single one of those items I would consider helpful. And every time I'd use one of those things, it would remind me how much I was loved. They were not just helpful, but comforting.

Remember, accepting and giving help comes in all forms. As the giver of help, pick the one that suits you best or what you see may be missing for the person in need.

- Are they struggling to eat? Bring them a smoothie to drink (packed with calories and protein) and a home cooked meal for the rest of the family.
- Do they need to get their mind off things? Bring them a good book (maybe the one you are reading right now).
- Do you have some extra funds in your account? Pay their electric or water bill so it's one less thing to worry about.
- Have an afternoon or evening to spare? Stop in and volunteer your time to help out wherever is needed.
- Are you making a grocery trip already this week? Pick up some extra items and drop it off at their house; who doesn't need more bread, milk and eggs?
- Are you exceptionally good with finances, HR items, yard work or fixing things around the house? Offer up your services. It would come at no cost to you, but could provide an abundance of help to the person in need.
- Are you a believer of Jesus? Add them to your prayer lists. There is power in prayer.

If you are the receiver of help and the one in need, don't be afraid to accept it. In tragic or difficult moments, others don't always know what exactly to do but they feel a desire to do something. They want to help their friend that is hurting. You're the friend. So just let go and let them.

CHAPTER 14

AN ANGEL NAMED JULIE

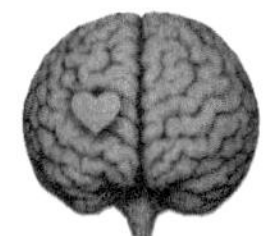

Once you learn to accept the help, there will come a point where you will have the opportunity to seek it out. In this instance, I am not referring to the help I mentioned in the previous chapter. This type of help is from nonprofit organizations or government funded agencies. As I mentioned before, I was amazed at all the connections that my very own friends and acquaintances had that I was completely unaware of prior to Sean's stroke. There are so many services out there to help you, it's just a matter of finding them. It can be very tedious and time consuming work, but I will let you know what I personally found helpful and what I discovered to be a waste of time. I'll inform you of my mistakes or misconceptions early on, so that you don't make the same ones and can skip right to the helpful ones. Hopefully my trial and error will only save you more time and headaches.

The first thing I did early on was start the process of applying for Social Security Disability Income (SSDI). I started this process about two weeks after Sean's stroke in early February. I had been told by many people that getting disability can be a long waiting game and more often than not, you are denied benefits the first time around, so it is best to start this process as soon as possible.

One of the brochures that The Stroke Care Manager from U of L Hospital gave me was a pamphlet advertising a company that offered "Free help with Disability Benefits." This particular company would interview you and then let you know based on the information you provided, if a legal representation would help your case. Kelly sat in with me while I did an initial call with the company. They did feel that getting an attorney would be beneficial and at the time, we both agreed this would be a good step to take as well. After all, I was feeling so overwhelmed with Sean's health and recovery that the thought of taking something off of my plate and giving it to a professional sounded wonderful. So they assigned me to a Disability Attorney based out of Tennessee, who agreed to take our case.

The phone call with my attorney's assistant was pretty straightforward. She explained the contract and answered any questions that we had. During that call, she was helpful. She explained that they only get paid if we win and the fee was $9,200 or 25% of his benefits awarded, whichever was less. Yes, it seemed like a lot of money but, at that time, I thought, *Well, that's money that I'm not expecting anyways, so I'm happy to pay that.* I signed the contract and proceeded to wait for my next steps.

Over the next couple of weeks, she would simply send me emails with links to fill out for the SSDI application or they'd request Sean's physician information. For the most part, I was doing the majority of the work. When I'd have a question, I would have to call multiple times or send multiple emails before I would get a response. Within a month of signing the contract, I started to regret my decision to go with this attorney. But I was stuck and contract bound to this law firm. Had I been taken advantage of in my vulnerable state and for lack of better words, screwed myself?

As the weeks went by and I learned more about the SSDI process and I was thinking clearer, I would have questions that the law firm simply would not or could not answer. I'm not sure which, as

I stopped getting responses altogether. Mind you, I never once communicated with the actual attorney assigned to me. Unfortunately, this is one of those instances in the early days that seemed a good idea but I quickly discovered it was a mistake. One that could have cost me a lot of money. I obviously couldn't go back in time and "unsign" the contract. But what options did I actually have?

While dealing with the not-so-helpful disability law firm, I was also receiving information on how Sean could qualify for different state government programs. The first one I heard about was Kentucky's Traumatic Brain Injury (TBI) Trust Fund, and I was encouraged to apply for it on Sean's behalf. It is open to all Kentucky residents, of all ages and income levels, who have a medically documented brain injury. It is offered through the state government and has nothing to do with Medicaid. The TBI Trust Fund was created to provide support to those with medically documented brain injuries through fines collected from DUI's and court costs. The trust fund is a payer of last resort and is designed to assist community-based resources in helping people with brain injuries maintain the highest quality of life possible.

During our long days at Frazier Rehabilitation, I had plenty of time to fill out the application, gather Sean's medical records and fax it all over to the TBI Trust office. You must be able to provide medical records from when the brain injury occurred, neurological evaluations, history and physical reports and medical consent forms. (Side note, I never had an issue with requesting the hospital or rehab to fax paperwork at the nurses station. Many of the business documents require a lot of faxing and they will do so at no charge. Taking the paperwork to a UPS Store, or somewhere similar, will charge you over $1 per page, so that adds up when you're faxing 100 page documents over to twenty different places. Take advantage of the facility you are living in. After all, it is your temporary home). I applied for the TBI Trust for Sean in mid-February and was found eligible by mid-March. It was overall a very quick and easy process and I'd highly recommend applying for this or a similar program in your state if you qualify.

Once he was made eligible, we were assigned a case manager that was located in our county of residence. Judy showed up to our home to meet with Sean and me. She greeted us with a friendly smile and was eager to tell us all about the TBI program. Sean had been approved for a trust amount of up to $15,000 per year, with a max of $60,000 in a lifetime. There are guidelines for how these funds can be used. They can be used for environmental modifications, companion or personal care, therapies or counseling services and respite care, among other things. The money cannot be used to cover medications, institutionalization, hospitalization, legal fees or any previous incurred debt or bill. Judy explained that for anything we were interested in, we simply submitted a request through her to be turned into the TBI Trust committee that meets once every three months. They will look over the paperwork and either approve or deny the requests.

I submitted a request immediately for handrails to be installed on our front and back porches and also going into our pool since he would probably be using that for therapy during the summer time. This required for me to gather quotes, a letter from his physician explaining the need for the handrails and a copy of the deed to our home. During the May meeting, our request was approved and we had new handrails installed in June. It was over $3,000 in home modifications that were completely covered by the trust. And those small improvements made such a huge difference in Sean's confidence and safety to go up and down the stairs.

The second program I heard about was the Kentucky Acquired Brain Injury Waiver, or ABI Waiver. There are other states that have some form of ABI Waiver, but most do not. The waivers will vary state to state on what they cover and how they function. ABI waiver programs are for adults with an acquired brain injury who can benefit from intensive rehabilitation services. The services are designed to help the participant re-enter the community and function independently. The Long Term Care ABI Waivers are for participants who have reached a plateau in the rehab level and require maintenance services to live safely in the community. Both of these waivers are funded through Medicaid and require you to apply for Medicaid, therefore require financial eligibility.

I applied for this waiver program mid February. Like the TBI Fund, it required an extensive application process and medical records to be faxed. I originally applied for the waiver using the assistance of a lady with a case management company, whose name was passed on to me from a friend. Although they had never worked with this particular case manager, she knew this was something important that I needed to get for Sean.

Within a month, Sean received the good news that he was accepted for the waiver program and a spot would be held for him for 60 days and I would have to apply for Medicaid during that time. I reached back out to the lady and I got very little help in return. I was left to kind of just figure the Medicaid application out on my own. My emotions were still extremely high during this time and feelings of overwhelm and this lack of help left me feeling lost and stuck, trying to understand what I needed to do.

It was about this time when the heavens parted and a lady named Julie fell straight out of the sky with her angel wings still intact and landed right in my arms. In reality, a massage guest gave me the name of an ex co-worker, who referred me to a State Brain Injury employee, who introduced me to a new ABI Case Management Company, who put me in contact with Julie. But it's just easier to say that an angel from heaven fell into my lap, because that is exactly who Julie became to me.

Julie is the Marketing Director at Caring Moore Homes and has more than 26 years of experience in the ABI, Medicaid and Disability. She was extremely knowledgeable about the Medicaid system, with a speciality in "holding your hand" during the entire process.

She was my kind of girl and exactly what I needed. I have no problems getting the job done, I just need someone to point me in the right direction. Julie reached out to me immediately and we scheduled a time to meet the following week at our house to go over the process. In the meantime, she emailed me an entire Medicaid Application Checklist of items that I would need to gather and have prepared when she arrived. Well, you already know I love a good checklist. This one was huge. I had to pull together every piece of financial information in my possession and even some I didn't have. All bills, motor vehicle values, pay stubs, retirement funds, value of home, bank statements, health insurance, life insurance, stocks and burial plots. And that's just to name a few (full list of required items in Chapter 19). It felt like everything but an actual blood sample was required. I proudly spent the time gathering all the info and placing it neatly into a folder to be ready for Julie when she arrived. Luckily, since I am an overall organized person, finding all the items was a little easier, but was still very time-consuming.

Julie arrived and I greeted her at the door. Like Judy with the TBI Trust, she seemed very energetic and bubbly but also ready to get to work. She introduced herself to Sean, who was sitting in his lounge chair, and proceeded to set up her computer at the kitchen table, put on her reading glasses and get down to business. I could tell that she knew her stuff and there was something about her that made me immediately trust her. Which was a comforting feeling seeing as how I didn't have a clue what I was doing and was handing her the value of every asset that we owned. She fingered through the thick folder of papers and entered information into her spreadsheet, while scanning copies of each and every document I provided. Every now and then, she'd ask for clarification and I scurried around in file drawers or looked stuff up on the computer to get her more details for her inquiries.

After more than an hour, she was ready to tell me her findings. She took her glasses off, placed her hand on mine and took a deep breath. There really wasn't any way to prepare myself for the wealth of information that was about to spew out of this angel's mouth. I'm sure in her mind she thought, "here goes nothing."

I recently tuned in to a short documentary called *Caregiving* on PBS. Paul Irving, Senior Advisor at the Milken Institute, made a profound statement in the show. He said, "Americans are not prepared for challenges of caregiving. Oftentimes, these things happen out of the blue. What you realize is that health, life, and casualty insurances don't cover these needs. So who is going to help you pay? The cost of caregiving is unbelievably high for many people and unaffordable for most. Medicare provides no caregiving support and Medicaid, which is a program that supports low income Americans, does provide limited support. So incredibly, more and more middle class Americans are forced to pay down to poverty so that they can qualify for Medicaid. That's a crazy system. It's a crazy system for them. It's a crazy system for our federal government."

Julie began explaining to me just that. The laws and guidelines of the crazy system. She went down her spreadsheet line by line showing me the value of each asset that was in mine and Sean's names. All the things and money that we have worked so very hard for. The peaks and valleys of our finances over the last two decades. Then came the rules of qualifying for Medicaid. I sat at the table and felt myself take a deep breath as well, preparing myself for what was to come. She took all of our assets and gave it a total value.

For simplicity purposes of explaining this, let's just say that those assets came to $100,000. That being said, this figure DOES NOT include the value of our home, the most expensive vehicle or our retirement savings. She took that $100,000 and divided it equally by two, giving myself $50,000 and Sean $50,000. To qualify for Medicaid, Sean cannot have more than $2,000 to his name at the end of any given month. That is the poverty level that Mr. Irving mentioned in the documentary.

So, the obvious question is, if he can only have $2,000, what do we do with the remaining $48,000? What you cannot do when applying for Medicaid, is give away money or assets. They can look back for a five year period to make sure there was not an inappropriate transfer of assets. Julie talked about the options of what you can do with the $48,000, one of which could be to pay down your home mortgage. But once that money is gone, it's gone, even if your house is paid down. You can't access that money again. So she continued on with what most of her clients choose to do.

Julie began explaining to me about a Special Needs Trust (SNT). A SNT is a legal arrangement that is designed to hold and manage money and property in an irrevocable trust — meaning, once created, cannot be changed, modified or terminated — for the benefit of a person with a disability without jeopardizing their eligibility for government benefits, such as Medicaid. It is a way to protect our assets and still allow Sean to qualify for Medicaid. Therefore, in this math equation, we would have to transfer $48,000 over to this trust, which also means we have to relinquish over all control of what we can spend that chunk of money on. This would now be in the hands of an attorney who we would have to ask and be given permission from to use any of that money moving forward.

I began glassing over as I tried to take in this information. I wasn't fully comprehending the magnitude of what I was feeling. Was she telling me I just had to give our money away? She continued on. The other side of this is that Sean cannot make more than $2901 per month. Any amount earned over $2901 would have to be transferred to a Qualified Income Trust (QIT), also called a Miller Trust. If you make more than that amount, you must set up a QIT to qualify for Medicaid long-term care benefits. This is another type of irrevocable trust that must be drawn up by an attorney. The monies that go into the QIT can only be used for specific, Medicaid-allowed expenses. Permitted uses of these funds can vary depending on if the recipient chooses to live in their own home versus a nursing facility. Julie also mentioned that you should keep in mind that the rules for a single person and a married couple are different. When you are married there is much more paperwork that has to be turned in since there are two people they are reviewing as a whole. If you are single your home is only exempt with a letter of intent to return home. Medicaid does not take into consideration what it will cost to keep that house, mortgage, monthly expenses, home owners insurance cost, and more.

I think after she went over everything, the look on my face was probably the look of defeat. I just felt so overwhelmed. I had grown to really hate that word as it seemed to be the adjective that described me every minute of every day. I tried so hard to take in everything she was telling me but it was just too much, and what was so great about Julie, is she could tell.

She closed up her computer, gave me an empathetic grin and said, "Why don't you take some time to think about everything. I'm going to email you over all of this. If you have any questions at all, don't hesitate to reach out. I'm here to help you and to help Sean." As she packed up her items and walked towards the door, she put her hand on Sean's shoulder. "It's going to be okay." She said while looking down at him. "I'm going to make sure you all are taken care of."

Julie allowed small feelings of comfort to creep in through the typical overwhelm. I walked her out and returned to the couch sitting next to Sean. My eyes immediately filled with tears, but I didn't let them fall. Yet. Sean has seen that worried look on my face countless times and this was no different.

"Were you listening?" I asked him quietly. I didn't want to cry but I could feel it filling up inside of me.

"A little." He managed to mumble back so I could understand him.

"I don't know what to do and I'm scared to death I'm going to make the wrong decision. I want what is best for you and your recovery, but I don't want to turn all of our money over. We worked too hard for it." And with that, the tears poured out of my eyes and down my face. And what was even more difficult is this was an exact situation that Sean and I would have talked over, discussed and made the decision together. Together. Something that was impossible to do now. All of the weight was on my shoulders and once again, I felt that lonely feeling. Sean was right there in front of me, yet I felt completely alone. Alone to make this huge decision.

I pleaded with him, "I don't know what to do and I need you right now." I curled up in his lap and put my tear-stained face on his chest, his left arm curling around me.

Sean looked at me and with all of his might and strength, he very slowly spoke these words to me. It was once again, mumbled, but I knew what he said. "I can't help you right now. Talk to your friends and take some time to think about it. You'll make the right decision." Aside from the one-armed hug, it was the best comfort he could provide me at that time. He knew this decision was big, but he wasn't able to comprehend and process the information Julie gave me in order to be helpful. He saw me hurting and worrying. And with that advice, I laid down on the couch and cried myself to sleep for a much needed afternoon reset.

I spent the next week going over the Medicaid information. I researched the SNT and QIT and sent Julie multiple follow-up emails, which she answered with great care and detail. I took Sean's advice and spoke to a couple of friends. I scheduled a meeting with the attorney that would draw up the SNT, who addressed all of my concerns and questions as well. And I prayed for guidance to make the best decision.

I felt so much better about everything after I gave myself time to take it all in and process the information myself. The weight didn't feel quite so heavy. Ultimately, I decided to move forward with setting up the QIT and SNT to apply for Medicaid in order to get the ABI waiver. I think what it came down to was writing out a pros and cons list. If I kept regular healthcare insurance for Sean, I was going to spend a small fortune to keep our same coverage and with basic healthcare, your insurance will only cover a certain amount of therapies per year. And limited therapies meant slower progress in his overall recovery. We would be limited and restricted. This would then start all over with a new deductible at the beginning of the calendar year. Anything above and beyond that coverage would have to be received through private pay. With the ABI Waiver, it will kick in once Medicaid no longer covers the therapies. So, as long as he is on the waiver, he can get an unlimited amount of therapies and counseling. He is also able to receive companion support, behavioral services, respite care and minor home modifications as needed. And with the exception of a monthly patient liability based on the recipient's income, these services would be at no cost.

By the end of March, after working closely with Julie, I realized I needed to terminate my relationship with the Tennessee Disability law firm. I was continuing to get very little response from them and was getting significantly more help from Julie, even with disability. Her angel wings continued to get bigger by the day! She had earned my trust fully and had already worked circles around the attorney. She was getting shit done and I was checking things off my list with her. She made me feel comfortable and safe, and in the midst of a lot of unknown emotions, I desperately needed that. She explained to me that, with a traumatic brain injury, you do not even need an attorney to file. It is very different from other physical issues or mental health.

"Either you have a brain injury or you don't. It's really that simple." Then she said, "I'll be your disability rep and I won't charge you a dime." Now, a halo was forming over her head to match the wings.

After inquiring about the charge that I could possibly incur for breaking my relationship with the Tennessee law firm, as the contract was not clear on that, they ended up sending me a termination letter. Which I replied with my own letter as well. Within a couple of weeks, I received a letter in the mail from both the law firm and social security stating that they still planned to petition to receive the $9,200 when I get approved for Disability. With an attached bill for the full six hours they had spent on my case. I'll go ahead and let you know that five of those hours I did myself. That sickening feeling filled my stomach. Did I just screw us? I didn't know what to do. I was simply following the advice given to me early on. At that time, it seemed like the right thing to do. If only I had met Julie while Sean was in the ICU.

With the help of Julie, Sean was approved for Disability, the first time, five months after applying. He would start receiving Social Security Disability Income immediately. Here's what I ended up learning through my experience when it comes to SSDI. You definitely don't need an attorney, but I do think you need a Julie, or a representative of some kind. The process is a lot to understand and navigate and it was a Godsend having her experience to guide me through it.

The other thing I learned? You cannot receive your first payment until five months after the event causing the disability. A disability attorney can only recoup their 25% or $9,200 payment from BACK PAY. That's right, back pay. So I realized quickly why I wasn't getting my questions answered in a timely manner from them. Pushing me off was going to get them paid. They didn't want me to get disability approval before the five months. So, lucky for me, I dodged a bullet. Julie worked at my pace, so there was no back pay, which meant there wasn't any money for the attorney to collect. So, that Tennessee law firm that billed me $9,200 for six hours of my own work, won't see a dime of Sean's disability.

Once SSDI was approved, Medicaid was approved three weeks later. I'm not going to lie to you, Medicaid was an absolute nightmare to deal with. You will absolutely want to have a representative helping you with Medicaid, or at least someone who is very knowledgeable with the process. It is extremely confusing to the point that at times, I was convinced they only wanted to push applicants to the limit of giving up. I would think everything was complete, only to have them request something else. Up until the last day, I was still running to the banks, DMV and making last minute mortgage payments to show the correct income for Sean in order to receive Medicaid.

I had a strict deadline to get the ABI Waiver for him, which was the only reason I was even pursuing Medicaid. Julie got me a 24-hour extension and with only eight hours left of the last day, we were able to get the approval. There is no way I could have done it without Julie fighting for me and advocating for Sean. Her experience and persistence paid off. Not to mention the many pep talks she would give me along the way when I was either about to have a breakdown or ready to throw in the towel. She never gave up and I can't thank her enough for that.

Per Julie, once approved for Medicaid, you will only have to complete an annual review moving forward (although technically they can audit whenever, just like any other government agency). For the annual review, you will need to furnish updated three months of all bank statements, your current award letter, and if you have any new assets or sold any assets over the last year. As long as there is a paper trail for all money that has gone out or come in it is usually pretty easy to do the renewal.

Literally the day after Medicaid was approved, I was setting up services with Sean's ABI case manager. He was able to continue with his speech, occupational and physical therapies and was set up with companion services. I could continue to go to work and I no longer had to rely on Mike, Karen and Kathy in order to do so. They could just be parents and grandparents again. And I didn't have to worry about Sean's safety while I was gone. All of the hard work was finally paying off and Sean was going to continue to get the care he needed for the best recovery possible.

If you've read this chapter in one setting, I'm sure your head feels like it's about to explode and I've only added to the overwhelmingness. Take a deep breath. Breathe in and slowly breathe out. Maybe wipe the tears streaming down your face and take one more deep breath for good measure. It's going to be okay.

Here are my takeaways when it comes to Disability and Medicaid. Outside of the health recovery of your loved one, these will be some of the biggest challenges to get through. It requires a lot of time, dedication and even research if you don't already have the materials readily available. In an ideal world, have your paperwork in order and everything you need before tragedy strikes. Power of Attorney and Living Wills are so important and, in the event of something happening, will make things much easier to navigate.

Looking back, based on my personal experience, I would file for Disability first, then Medicaid and then the ABI Waiver or whatever is similar in your state. When I asked Julie the same question, she told me it really depends on the individual. Each person's situation is different. I would suggest filing for disability as soon as possible. Something to keep in mind is they will not make an initial decision until at least 90 days after injury. All doctor's appointments and therapy sessions you can schedule after day 91 is what they are going to be reviewing. They will gather all therapy and office visit notes from appointments after that date. They want to know where that individual is in their functioning day 91 forward. They don't really care where they were before that day. A lot of families need to start getting their materials together for Medicaid as soon as possible as well. Many may have to go through the process of getting Power of Attorney (POA) or guardianship in order to access employer and retirement account information, among other things. Sean and I did not have these things and I was only able to get so far before needing a POA or guardianship.

I ran into a problem because I was told by the medical staff early on that Sean wasn't in good enough health to give me POA, but when I spoke to an attorney was told he wasn't bad enough to get guardianship. So, things came to a halt for me until Sean was able to improve enough for an attorney to set up a POA in order for me to continue gathering the information needed. Me just being his wife only got me so far. In hindsight, definitely set up your POA, Living Will and/or Living Trust early on before you actually are going to need it. It will save you the extra headache.

Get a representative when applying for both Disability and Medicaid. It will help preserve your sanity. Ideally, find a Julie. Or better yet, find Julie herself if you're in the state of Kentucky. You can also reach out and call any of the ABI Case Managers to assist you with this. Although I did not personally use them, I've heard positive things about stroke survivors using Allsup, National Social Security Disability Representatives. A lot of times their services can be provided free of charge through the employer's Long Term Disability if they qualify.

There will be multiple times during the first year where you absolutely will have to give yourself time to process. There is so much information being thrown your way and you're not always going to be on your A-Game to take it all in. Don't make any rash decisions. Do your own research, ask for advice and don't be afraid to ask all the questions. The clearer you are about everything, the more confident you will feel when the time comes to make the decision.

CHAPTER 15
I AM NOT ALONE

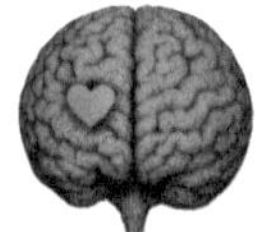

was surrounded by friends and family throughout the time after Sean's stroke, yet a part of me still felt so alone. Mike and Karen were staying at our house half of the week. Kathy was over several times a week as well. The Homegirls would show up in a moment's notice if I needed them for an "emergency cocktail hour" and I had others who planned dinner outings weeks ahead of time. Sean was here with me and making baby steps of progress each and every day.

So, why did I still feel so lonely? I talked to my therapist about this of course, but even she couldn't actually relate. She could only give me advice based on textbooks she read or other patients she had in the past that went through a similar situation. I didn't have anyone in my life that really knew what I was going through. The day to day struggles, how I was really feeling, the loss I felt, the frustrations I was experiencing, and even why I'd get so excited simply because Sean moved his arm a fraction of a centimeter. My life was so different than it had been a year before. While everyone else continued on with their lives, I was still very much adjusting to mine.

Melissa suggested joining some online support groups to me while Sean was still in the hospital. At the time, I wasn't ready and she knew that but was planting a bug in my ear. There were several in-person support groups that Frazier of U of L Hospital offered, both for myself and Sean. At that time, the thought of adding one more destination to my weekly schedule seemed impossible. There didn't feel like enough hours in the day as it was to take care of everything, so for me, I preferred the online route anyways.

Once we were home and settled in, I decided to look around on Facebook and found a page for the caregivers of stroke survivors. I clicked the "Join Group" button and immediately I was added into the group. It didn't take long for me to realize that group just wasn't for me. I was seeking support and encouragement, but instead I was reading doom and gloom stories. Many of the members were posting about being at their breaking points. I felt like all I saw was constant negativity and giving up mentalities. Don't get me wrong, I can fully comprehend how this life of being a caregiver can get the best of you. The person you are caring for is simply not the same person you knew before. They're just…different. A lot of the members in this group had been going through this for years so they're current experiences were the same, but also very different from mine.

I was and am a new stroke survivor's wife. I wanted to focus on the positives, the accomplishments and the goals that were being achieved! I still had hope. I wasn't in burn out mode or ready to throw in the towel. But a lot of these posts were dimming my hope and my light. I could quickly feel myself going to a dark place and I knew I needed to get out of the group fast. It just wasn't a good fit for me at that moment. I stuck around for a few months giving the group plenty of opportunities to change my mind, but ultimately decided to leave the group. Shortly after that, in true social media algorithm form, a suggested group popped up in my Facebook feed. "Stroke Survivor's Wives Only." I was intrigued at the fact that this group was more specific to my personal role and decided to try again by giving them a chance. Maybe it would be exactly what I was looking for. I clicked the request to join button and was prompted to immediately answer several questions; confirm you are the caregiver to your husband, when was the stroke, what type of stroke was it? Do you agree to post an intro within seven days of being admitted into the group?

Wow, very thorough. I thought. I already felt better about this group. I answered the questions and clicked agree and waited for an administrator to accept me in the group. Within 24 hours, I was officially a member and began writing up my required introduction post. I included pictures of Sean and I both pre and post stroke. I was welcomed with open arms, kind words of encouragement and a guaranteed judgement-free zone. But there was one particular comment that stood out to me.

A lady stated, "Welcome to the sisterhood that no one wants to be a part of." That greeting just spoke volumes and really stuck with me, even to this day. She was right. I didn't want to be a part of this group. I didn't want this curve ball that life threw my way. Things were going fine before. I didn't want to be friends with these strangers, to know exactly what they were all feeling and going through. In reality, I was part of this sisterhood whether I wanted to be or not. And that one comment on my very first post in that group, was the reality check that I don't think I fully faced until then. I was an official member of the "Stroke Survivor's Wives Club."

Over the months and days, I realized I was really leaning into this elite group of women. I, all of a sudden, didn't feel so lonely. There was, unfortunately, an entire mass of women I could relate to. I found that when I'd read a story about their Stroke Survivor Husband (abbreviated to SS or SSH), I'd think "Sean did the same thing today!" These women were real and relatable. We share our own stories about how we became Stroke Survivor Wives. I'd learn about all the different types of strokes out there; ischemic, hemor-rhagic, TIA and the different effects that the strokes can cause. Some SSH can still walk and talk, but cognitively they'd really be struggling. Their personalities may be different or they were meaner or more sensitive. Other SSH were cognitively there, but were still completely wheelchair or bed bound. Some I'd read about, then wish Sean was doing as good as Ken, somebody else's SSH. He was only three months from his stroke and was already driving again and going to the grocery store and back to work. Other times, Sean would be miles ahead of another SSH. Their wives were still having to help them go to the bathroom or they refused to do therapies.

I'd feel especially closer to the women whose husbands had the same type of stroke and struggles as Sean. Then we could compare notes and it would give me that hope again that I cling on to for Sean's recovery. The milestones and timeframe would be very similar so it gave me something to strive for. I'd often even share these stories with Sean to give him hope too.

"Bill had the same stroke as you and he is now driving! And he's in his 60s!"

"John has aphasia too, but he's been able to go back to work!"

The ages of all the SS's and their wives were all over the place and ranged over five decades. Some are couples in their 70s and 80s with grandchildren and some as young as 30s with small children at home. We are all in different stages of our lives where usually we'd have nothing in common. However, because of one tragic event that chose to come into our lives, we all have one big thing in common. We're caregivers, mothers and employees. We are phys-ical therapists, speech coaches and teachers. We're chauffeurs, maids and home maintenance workers. We're Stroke Survivor's Wives.

There's always a variety of topics posted on the page, as well. It is a place to vent and not be judged. You can freely share how exhausted you are or that you want to curl up in a ball and cry. Or maybe you just want somebody to understand how you're all out of patience and if your SSH asks for one more thing, you may lose it. Or that you've lost friends and family that don't come to visit anymore and feel like you've just been left behind. And if you do make those posts, not only are you not judged for the things that others outside the Sisterhood may think are cruel or mean, but you're met with compassion, empathy and understanding. You're not told "how strong you are" because we already hear that enough from everyone else. Instead of "I can only imagine," you're met with "me too," "I feel the same," and "it's okay to stand up for yourself." You're built up to feel strong, even though you feel weak. You are made to feel alive, even though you feel so tired. You feel supported through the defeat and hope through the change.

It has also been a place for great celebration. Not everyone can comprehend the difficulty of what it takes for someone that has experienced a stroke or similar disability to relearn how to do such simple tasks. But this sisterhood does. Heart emojis and congratulatory words are expressed when a SSH takes five steps on his own, or can touch his nose again or can wiggle a finger. Some are even bigger achievements of going on a trip, attending a large event or doing something around the house. There is praise and happiness shared throughout. And even though I can get these same responses from my own friends and family, the women in this group really know and understand the magnitude of these very significant milestones. And it feels really great to share it with them and get such positive responses.

I've also been able to lean on them for advice. From fashion advice on finding stylish clothes that are also easy to get on and off to the best non-alcoholic beverages on the market. Sometimes it's learning about new devices or treatments that help with the recovery process. I've been educated on walking devices, botox treatments and AFOs (Ankle Foot Orthotic), all of which I have eventually gotten for Sean. It's just been a wealth of helpful information.

Even though each of our stories are a little different, these women and I are all still very much the same. We are overwhelmed and often feel unseen and unappreciated. However, we lift one another up and cheer each other on. We are all running the same marathon and we have the same goal. Our eyes are on the finish line and we want to cross over (preferably in one piece and with our sanity intact)! We have fight and grit. We are tired and heavy but the sweat and tears that cover our bodies will keep us pushing forward. The love we have for our husbands, the love I have for Sean, keeps me going. I am determined that we will conquer this obstacle and maybe even be better people for it on the other side. According to the Stroke Awareness Foundation, 1 in 5 Americans will suffer a stroke in their lifetime and a stroke occurs every 40 seconds. That means there are a lot of people out there that know what Sean and I are going through. It's just a matter of finding them.

If you're facing a similar situation, you are not alone either. I really encourage you to find your own support system when you are ready. For me, it wasn't immediately. I waited several months, mostly because I had to accept the fact I was in a position that I needed that support and that I even belonged in these groups. I had to move past denial and replace it with acceptance. There are always plenty of in-person support groups that you can attend by yourself or with your Stroke Survivor. If in-person isn't your preferred method, social media provides so many online groups out there. Some can be attended through a zoom call and others through messaging online. Even if you don't participate in those groups but only read or listen to what others are saying, I promise you will feel more understood and less alone. Also, once I realized how helpful my wives group was for me, I began encouraging

Sean to find his own online support group. He is now a part of his own stroke survivor groups, communicating with others that know exactly what he is going through and how he feels. Because I don't know how he feels as much as he doesn't know how I feel. We all need to find the support groups that work the best for us. We may feel lonely at times, but we are far from being alone.

CHAPTER 16
AMBIGUOUS GRIEF

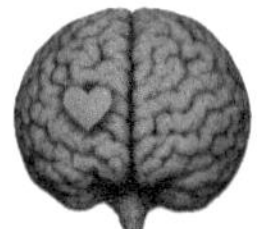

We have probably all experienced grief at some point in our lives. I remember going to my first funeral when I was around eight years old. It was my great-grandmother who passed. The room was filled with the scent of old people and floral arrangements, which masked together to make an exceptionally intense perfume aroma. The room was filled with quiet murmurs and sniffles from the tears being shed. It was a confusing situation for my young brain to understand. I wasn't feeling much emotion myself, but the room was telling me that I should be sad. As one gets older, we have the unfortunate circumstance of attending more and more funerals for the ones we love. The great grandparents turn into grandparents, which then turn into parents. And that's assuming it goes in that order. Each one gets a little harder and you quickly become one of the people in the corner murmuring and sniffling, versus the small child running around wildly through the corridors of the funeral home.

In a perfect world, knowing that everyone's human lives will end at some point, everyone would live to eighty, ninety or hundred. But we all know that isn't the case. The heart and body learns to deal with grief and their own ways of mourning, and can often depend on who it is that is passing on. The heart tends to break a little differently when you have to let go of someone young. You're obviously grieving for the loss of that person, but you're also grieving for the tragedy of what could have been and the life they could have had. Living in the "what ifs" can tear a person apart. I'm sure that is the case with the unimaginable death of a young friend or a child. The different kind of emptiness that one must feel losing a child, no matter your age. It's just not part of the natural progression of life and no one should have to endure that type of pain of burying their child. Seeing the pain that Kathy went through letting go of Chris, her only child, at the age of 21. It's gut wrenching. So much life ahead of him. So many great things that could have been. And Chris's friends felt similar feelings. Racing thoughts of 'life is short and nothing is promised,' We're not invincible like one thinks they are in their teens and twenties. Tragedy doesn't discriminate and death comes for everyone. It's just a matter of when.

I've found it very interesting how people deal with grief when losing someone. There's the basic guideline of the "five stages of grief," described by psychiatrist Elisabeth Kubler-Ross. Denial, anger, bargaining, depression and acceptance. People can move back and forth between them, skip some, and revisit others over and over again. But how you deal with grief doesn't mean that others deal with it the same way. There's no right or wrong way and everyone can be different. Some move on quickly "because that's what their loved one would want them to do." Others may never fully move on. It's important to allow the individual to grieve in their own way and in their own time.

Sometimes, grief doesn't come in the form of physically losing someone to death. I've, unfortunately, dealt with the circumstance of losing people in my life due to a downfall of the relationship that just couldn't be reconciled. It was ultimately best to go our separate ways. But did I grieve that relationship? Yes, I did. It honestly didn't feel much different than if I had lost them to death.

In some circumstances it felt the same as if they had passed on. I went through a lot of those five stages, especially anger, depression and acceptance. Acceptance being the hardest because I couldn't wrap my brain around losing a relationship that was once so close.

Then there was Sean's stroke. Another kind of grief. Ambiguous grief. I first heard the term in my Stroke Survivor's Wives group. I had definitely felt the feelings, but didn't know it actually had a name, and that so many others were experiencing the same thing. Ambiguous grief is grieving someone who is still there, which in a sense is similar to my failed relationships for those still earthside. Although my past experience didn't make this any easier. Mostly because it was different in the sense that we didn't choose the change. We were happy with our lives and looking forward to the future.

Ambiguous grief refers to the emotional pain experienced when a loved one is lost without a clear resolution, such as when they are physically absent but psychologically present, or vice versa. This type of grief complicates the mourning process because it lacks closure and condolences. It can leave you feeling confused and stuck, with no ending in sight. When I learned about this term, it took me back to that day when we moved Sean into inpatient rehab. That horrible day when Mike and Karen had to leave me in that large, empty room by myself having a full on breakdown. But that's the thing, I wasn't by myself. Sean was in the room with me, yet I felt so alone. His body was there but he, my husband Sean, was not. The tears I was crying that day were tears of grief. I was mourning the fact that my husband was alive right there next to me, but couldn't console me like he would have done so quickly in the past. He usually couldn't take seeing me cry. Yet there he was, laying in the bed while I sat in the corner. He couldn't hug me or tell me it was going to be okay. Even when he finally did come to, his consoling felt different. It felt emptier, with little emotion. He was somewhere in there, but very hard to find.

Ambiguous grief is cruel. For myself, I find it follows the roller coaster symbolism, similar to the amusement park ride that my emotions have been on. One day, grief being at an all time high, feeling like life will never be the same. Or the person you sit and have a conversation with doesn't feel like the same person you've known and loved for years prior. This horrible thing showed up and stripped all of that away from them. He's quiet when he used to talk my ear off. He's distant when he used to always touch me. And he's sad when he used to always be the life of the party. It's like I'd look at him and there was something that would be…missing. He's breathing and alive, but will also look at me with a blank stare and confusion. Trying to form the words and sentences. Trying to piece together the mayhem going on in his injured brain.

Then the amusement park ride peaks at the top of a hill. Things aren't so bad on these days. I started to feel as if we were going to make the most of what we still have. We're watching a video and laugh simultaneously at a joke. Conversations slowly don't feel so one sided and he is participating. People will come to visit and he's happy to see them. He can look at me and I can tell he still loves me and then he'll even tell me so. Up and down, up and down, up and down.

Part of this process is also grieving for the me who is also gone. Whether I like it or not, I've changed since Sean's stroke. In some ways, I'm stronger. Like superwoman, strong. I feel like going through this has set me up to get through just about anything life throws at me. But I am also more on edge, anticipating the next scary thing that's bound to happen. It's going to, just a matter of when. I stay more anxious than I ever have before. With all the things I've been through in my life, I've never really had to deal with anxiety until now. I'd have small spurts of it, but it would go away fairly quickly. Now, my anxiety is always there. Some days it's a rain cloud over my head that doesn't want to go away and other days it stays more at a distance. But it's always there.

Ambiguous grief is also feeling the grief of what was and what could have been. Our life together was pretty great for the most part. Sure, we did our fair share of bickering and disagreeing as most married couples do, but overall it was a pretty fantastic life. We were dancing through life, both literally and figuratively. We had one son successfully moving through college, living his best life and the other with a flourishing social life and raw, musical talent that some people would give anything to have. And most importantly, both boys were healthy. And Sean and I both were healthy, until we weren't. Until that stroke came in and took it all away in mere seconds.

Remember that evil side of social media I mentioned before? It reared its ugly head to me the summer after Sean's stroke. All of the posts of family vacations and couples trips. I would scroll through picture after picture of beautiful beaches, breathtaking sunsets, mountain views and historical monuments. Families snuggled up in pictures with big smiles on their faces. Children running around with friends and couples drinking wine on some magical vineyard in California or Venice, Italy. Just a year ago, those were my pictures being posted. My pictures of parasailing over the ocean and jet skiing on the waves. My pictures of meeting up with friends that moved to Florida to have dinner overlooking the ocean. My pictures of going to a Major League Baseball stadium as a family.

There was no posting these pictures now. Instead my posts were updates on Sean's health, not of fancy vacations. Some may view this as jealousy, and yes, it may be a little bit of that, too. But it's also grief. I'm happy for my friends that get to take these trips. I'm sure they worked hard to be able to go on them. But I'm also mourning the fact that we cannot do that. And I don't know when we will be able to do that again. I even convinced myself we could go somewhere just the two of us, close by, for a long weekend, after viewing these social media posts. I got on Airbnb, hoping to find a cute little retreat or cabin where we could go relax. It would still be a lot of work for me, but I thought it could be something fun to do together. I put in a variety of dates and locations in the search bar. Up popped 728 options fitting the criteria I was looking for. I opened up the filter and clicked on the option for handicap accessible. 728 quickly decreased to two options. That's right. Two. My hopefulness for a surprise getaway was met with immediate despair and grief. I closed the application and put down my phone. I felt so defeated and just really sad. I have yet to open the Airbnb app again since that day.

Last year, Sean and I took a trip of a lifetime to Greece. It was a vacation we dreamed about, but were never sure would actually happen. Then Sean found out he was going to Poland for work, so we took advantage of his paid airfare and tagged on a vacation in Greece. It was unbelievable. Every aspect of it was just a total dream. Our relationship grew closer over that trip too. We cherished every moment and mentioned multiple times how grateful we were to be there and sharing this experience with one another. We knew then how lucky we were. I feel it more now, seeing where we are today.

When we got home, we dreamed about all the other places we wanted to visit around the world together and of maybe even taking the boys somewhere overseas. We wanted to learn about other cultures and countries. Italy, Switzerland, New Zealand, Ireland and Australia. The possibilities were endless. And now, I don't know if we'll ever be able to do a trip like that again. That once-in-a-lifetime trip may have been just that. Once in a lifetime.

I've always enjoyed walking outside. It's a stress reliever for me and I love being out in the open air. Sean hates walking. A neighborhood walk has always been very boring to him with not enough to look at. But what he does enjoy doing is being out in nature. He loves yard work, planting and caring for flowers and plants and even dabbling in some gardening. I, not so much.

We finally figured out how to combine the two things though a few years back. We started finding hiking trails in local parks and nearby vacation destinations. We loved it. There were sights for him to see and I was out getting exercise. We'd talk the whole time and admire the animals and flowers we'd see along the trails. Sometimes we'd put some music on to accompany our adventures but we'd also like the peacefulness that nature alone would bring. It had become our thing. We even bought each other hiking boots for Christmas that following year. Now, I don't know when or if we'll be able to hike together again. Grief for another thing that was and may never be again.

That's the thing with ambiguous grief that's like normal grief. Others will be there initially, offering up help or assistance or a shoulder to cry on. But their lives continue to move forward, while yours remains still. Or at least it's moving so slow, it feels like it might as well be sitting still. For me, it's circling around Sean's stroke, and it gets to call the shots on what we can and can't do now. It's in control. And maybe for you, it's dementia that's in control. Or cancer or multiple sclerosis or Parkinson's disease. Or is it actually in control? It may feel that way on some days or most days. I think that's where that fifth step of grief comes in. Acceptance.

I went through denial almost immediately. Pure shock of the situation. This can't be real. I'm numb so it must be a nightmare. Why Sean? Why me? Why our boys? It isn't fair. That quickly turned to anger. Why didn't Sean go to the doctor when I asked him to? Why did God have to punish him this way for not going to the doctor? It isn't fair. Bargaining with God. Depression sinking in. First with me, then with Sean. Is this really our reality now? Is this what the next fifty years will be like? I'm so heavy and exhausted. It isn't fair. Now I've arrived at acceptance. Which is still a work in progress if I'm being honest. But I feel like that's a good thing. I haven't accepted things because I don't feel like it's actually over, whereas regular grief, unlike the ambiguous kind, is more finalized. This isn't our final destination.

I may start accepting that our dreams to backpack across Europe won't happen, but that doesn't mean that I can't create new dreams. My new personal dream is to become an advocate for other stroke survivors and their loved ones. To have my book become a useful tool to help them navigate this unknown path. It's scary, but it's a little less scary if you have someone to help you through it.

My dream for Sean is that he will be able to piece together words and find his voice again. So that he may speak to others about men's health or to other stroke survivors and give them hope in this new life. Sean's new personal dream is to be able to drive again and mow his own lawn. We still have our dreams to travel and see the world, but we'll just have to tackle those trips differently than we did before. There won't be hiking the foothills of Mount Tibidabo, but maybe cruising through the Mediterranean or Hawaii. We can still grieve for what could have been, but accept what is our reality and dream of what could be. Because those new dreams can still be endless.

CHAPTER 17
CHICKENBURGER

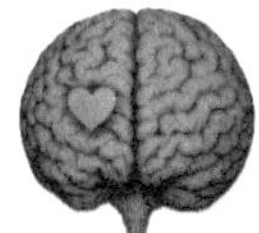

troke Brain. It's a common phrase used in the stroke community. It can be said when a stroke survivor is having memory issues that they've never had before. Or maybe it is used to describe the extra process time it takes to think of what needs to be said or done. Or maybe it is the difficulty that they have when expressing their emotions, or lack thereof. Sometimes caregivers will also experience seeing a change in their stroke survivor's personality causing them to say or do things that were very unlike their pre-stroke self. Stoke brain is not necessarily an actual medical diagnosis, but more of a term used when dealing with stroke recovery and everything that comes along with that. It can definitely be challenging for both the survivor and caregiver, often causing emotions to rise when dealing with certain situations. On the flip side, it can also provide a tense situation with some comedic relief.

One weekend, during Sean's inpatient stay at Frazier Rehabilitation, he lay in his hospital bed with the family surrounding him. We had just gotten over the hump of his refusal to take in enough calories in order to get through his therapies and heal. We had been tracking everything he was eating and drinking in the hopes that a feeding tube would not have to be put back in. It was that piece of cheesecake from the Cheesecake Factory that was the positive turning point for him and opened up his eyes and stomach to all the foods he could eat again. Landon was in town, visiting from college, that weekend so the whole family was hanging out in his room. The rumbles of everyone's stomachs sparked the conversation of what to get for dinner. Hospital cafeteria food was no longer an option.

Sean was pretty alert that particular day and was sitting up attempting to converse with all the visitors. We began discussing what to get to eat. Sean chimed in with his own thoughts. Except during that time, when it was early on into his aphasia and speech therapy, it was more of a combination of charades and Pictionary when attempting to figure out what he was trying to communicate. Thank goodness for those time periods in my life I was addicted to the Game Show Network because it really came in handy with my guessing skills.

We brought out the white board and marker, a picture chart the therapist had left in the room and was in a full on guessing game of "yes" and "no" questions. He wanted a chickenburger and white chocolate milkshake. He was adamant that we were correct on our guesses and was vigorously nodding his head yes. We guessed correctly what Sean was saying, but we still had to translate it into what he was actually trying to say. It provoked a lot of cheering when answers were guessed correctly and laughter when the correct answer emerged. It was apparently a chickenburger. After continued guessing, we were able to conclude that he wanted a Chick-fil-a chicken sandwich and a vanilla milkshake, and that is exactly what he got. That was our first experience with stroke brain.

Although it has slowly gotten better, Sean's communication struggles caused by his aphasia and stroke brain still continue to this day. He often will yell out "MOM" when I am in the other room. Karen hasn't been around in days and I'm the only other person in the house. The thing is, I am who he actually wants, not Karen. But when he opens his mouth, "Mom" is the word that comes out. I often will just hang out outside of the door, waiting to see what he will say next. Sometimes, "Mom" will come out again if I haven't responded quickly enough, but more often than not, I hear him let out a big sigh, which is usually a sigh of frustration with himself.

Then he'll yell "BABE!" I'll pop around the corner with a grin, proud that he was able to realize that he said mom when he wanted me, processed that that was not my name, thought of my correct name (Babe in this case, as it is what we've called one another since we were dating), and then said my correct name. Believe it or not, it takes him a lot of brain power and focus to make all those connections. He will even look at me at times and say, "Sorry, it's because of the stroke."

The first time he said that I died laughing. Of course he's calling me mom because of the stroke. He'd laugh too and would often use that phrase as an excuse for many things, stroke related or not. A lot of grace is given to him in those moments though and I try to stay patient to allow him to make the corrections on his own time. It's not unusual for him to ask for more salt in his coffee too, which on the days where my patience runs a little thinner, I'm tempted to do exactly that! But I keep myself in check and just add in the sugar instead.

We've all met those people before that forget to use, or choose not to use, what a lot of us refer to as their "filter." You know that part of the brain that allows us to think before we speak. Or there's things we want to say or do, but our brain's filter allows us not to react and instead, keep it to ourselves. Well, the location of the brain where Sean's stroke was, affected that filter as it does for many stroke survivors. There was a lot of eye rolling early on. If he thought something was stupid or he didn't agree with it, those eyes would go all the way in the back of his head, oftentimes simultaneously combined with a deep, irritating sigh. It was like having a bratty teenager all over again. At first, I was unsure how to approach him since he wasn't a teenager, but a grown man. But a stroke can tend to reset the brain and new neural pathways have to be created. This is obviously the case when learning to walk and talk again, but it is also the case for how to appropriately act and react to everyday situations. Over time, he increasingly gets better with dealing with these types of things and the eye rolling has become filtered again.

There also seems to be zero patience. Not just with Sean, but with other caregivers I've spoken with. If he wants something, food, the AC turned down, the lights turned off, he wants it done immediately. It doesn't matter if I'm running around doing ten other things. There was one day I was starting to prepare dinner, changing over a load of clothes and plunging a toilet (that he was responsible for clogging), which in turn had me cleaning the toilet.

While washing my hands multiple times, he says "Babe?"

"Yes?" I responded in a rush since I was frazzled by everything going on at the same time.

"Can you get me some chips?"

These are those moments you reach deep down into your soul to ask God not to allow you to spout off what you really want to say. In other words, I was using my filter. The nicest thing I could come up with was, "No, not right now."

Luckily, he accepted my answer. I found over time that at first, I would never say "no." I simply would drop what I was doing and get him what he wanted. He needed me and I felt the urge to be there for anything and everything the instant he requested it. But as time passes and another day comes and goes, it can feel like Groundhog Day. I decided to change some of my "yes" replies to "nos." It allowed me to feel a little more in control of myself, instead of someone just spinning in place. He was going to have to either wait for the chips until I got a moment, or if he wanted them badly enough, he could get up and get them. For him though as it is probably the case with so many, I think they are capable of getting what they need, but the time it takes them to get it takes much longer than just asking the caregiver or spouse. But by making them wait and teaching patience, it actually can make them become more independent which is a goal we all want to achieve. I will admit, this is still a continued work in progress. I have by no means mastered this part. We both still have a lot to learn and a long way to go.

Bossiness is another great virtue of a stroke survivor (cue sarcasm). Seeing as how he can't do a lot of the things he used to do, we all now get told the correct ways to do things, all while being critiqued. Driving with the GPS on to a destination is accompanied with Sean pointing to the lane we should be in, or the direction to go or the street to turn on. We are given a strict list of instructions of when and how to water the flowers in the back yard or how to empty the filter in the pool. He will watch us from the window and we'll be graded on our performance the moment we walk back in the house. Bossiness can definitely be a lot to take in. On the other hand, it's impressive that he even remembers a lot of these things.

It is also very common after a stroke to have emotional changes. One of my fears, when Sean was in the ICU and intubated, was that when he woke up, he'd be a totally different person. Would he be the same man that I fell in love with, who I've chosen to build my life with? I've read other stories and talked to other women whose husbands have turned mean, causing them to say things out of character, have a hateful demeanor, regular outbursts and just generally taking the anger inside them out on their loved ones. I imagine that some of these reactions may be another part of stroke brain.The mental struggle of simply dealing with and accepting this new way of life.

In the year since his stroke, there have only been two instances where Sean acted very out of character. Almost like temporarily he left his body and someone else jumped in. We had been home for a couple of months and were still adjusting to our new routines. He had been, what I thought at the time, lazy all day lying in his lounge chair watching movies. I, per usual, had been running around like a chicken with my head cut off. I was running to meetings, making phone calls, and taking care of the house. It was shower time, which as I said before is really a tiring feat for both of us. He had started using his cane to walk some, so I suggested he walk to the bathroom instead of using his wheelchair. He looked straight at me as he transferred himself over to the electric wheelchair and turned it on, which made a beep noise indicating it was ready to start moving.

"Come on babe. You've been sitting all day. Why don't you try to walk?"

"No," he responded bluntly.

Austin was in the room and he shot a quick glance over to me, like "What now, mom?"

I tried to compromise with him in a calming tone. "Alright, if you don't want to walk all the way to the bathroom, at least walk to me in the kitchen. Come on, you've got this!"

At that simple request, Sean piped off with what I can only assume was a full out cussing session, calling me every name in the book and telling me all the reasons why he didn't want to walk even one step. Although I understood little of what he said, it was clear from his tone exactly what he meant. I was completely taken back, and so was Austin. Sean always taught the boys to be respectful, especially to women, so Austin seeing this behavior coming from his dad really shocked him. We didn't even talk to one another that way even behind closed doors.

This wasn't my Sean. Here I was, at my wits end, doing everything and with a lot of patience and now I was being talked to this way! There is no way this would have been acceptable had he not had the stroke. Although, he also would have never talked to me that way if he hadn't had the stroke. I got him in the shower and never said a word, only held back tears. I think I was hurt more than anything. I stepped out of the room for a moment once he was safely in the shower. I contemplated saying anything to him.

Austin came into the room with a concerning look. "Mom, are you okay? Are you mad at Dad?"

"Yes, I am Austin. Do you think I was asking too much of him?" After all, I didn't know what I was doing. It was trial and error and I was just learning as I went.

"No, I don't think you were. I'm not sure why he got so mad." He was concerned and worried. You could see it in his eyes.

I went back into the bathroom and began to help him get out of the shower and dressed. I still couldn't even look at him, but said very directly in a quiet voice, "I'm doing a lot for you and you need me, but I won't be talked to that way. You cannot talk to me that way again." The hurt I was still feeling made tears stream down my cheeks as I spoke. I knew he couldn't help it, but it didn't make it hurt any less.

"I'm sorry babe," he said back to me. I looked up at him. He was hurting too. He didn't mean to talk to me that way, but he did. It's like he was trying to comprehend the situation as well. I have to remind myself in these instances that he is still functioning with a brain injury. As time passed since that incident, he has not snapped at me again. Not once. I think he is reteaching himself to "think before he speaks."

It is very easy to get frustrated with your SS. But remember, they are frustrated with themselves too. Imagine not feeling like yourself, but not being able to do anything about it. You are working and putting in the effort, but sometimes it feels impossible to accomplish things that used to be second nature. It would be incredibly hard. I really try to remind myself that every day. I am going through a hard time, but so is Sean.

Yelling at him or losing my patience isn't going to get us anywhere. I want to move forward, not in circles. My brain is the one without injury, therefore, the responsibility falls more on me. Now, don't get me wrong. That doesn't mean that your SS should be able to get away with murder, but it does mean it may take them longer to do things because extra time has to be spent to process it. Or they are bossy because they have taken pride in doing things on their own their whole life, but now depend on others to do it for them and to do it right. They are struggling every day to adjust and live this new life to the best of their ability. And I can guarantee they will be able to accomplish that better with love and support by their side. I came across this passage by Yvonne Kent Pateras that was really eye opening for me and put things into perspective on what a person with a brain injury struggles with on a daily basis.

"Living with a brain injury isn't the same every day - it changes, just like traffic lights. Some days are easier, and some days are overwhelming.

Green zone: These are the "good" days. Someone with a brain injury might seem almost like their old self - they can work, do chores, laugh, and even enjoy social events. But even on these days, it still takes more effort than it looks.

Orange zone: These are the "struggle" days. It feels like treading water - managing, but it's hard. Someone may be able to smile, chat or show up for things, but inside, it's exhausting. It takes all their energy just to keep going.

Red zone: These are the really tough days. It feels like drowning. Even simple things - like taking a shower, holding a conversation or being around people - can feel impossible. On these days, they may need to stay quiet, rest or be alone just to cope.

The important thing to understand is: people with brain injuries don't always look sick. They can sometimes smile, work or socialize, and other times they can't do even the smallest things. This doesn't mean they're lazy or not trying - it means their brain is fighting an invisible battle every day.

So, if someone you know has a brain injury, please be patient, don't judge, and don't expect them to "prove" how unwell they are. Their strength is in surviving each day, whether it's green, orange or red."

I read this passage to Sean, curious to see if this is how he felt. It was an immediate and resounding "YES!" If I find myself losing patience, getting frustrated or wanting to scream, I do just that. But I really try not to do it to Sean or *at* Sean. He's going through a lot. But so am I and I don't think that should be pushed to the side just because I'm not the one with the brain injury. That's when I turn to a homegirl, or set up a meeting with my therapist, or take a walk around the block. It's important for the stroke survivor to know that you have a lot on your plate too. And you need their patience as much as they need yours.

We sat in the living room together one evening, as we had grown accustomed to doing, Sean in his lounge chair and me on the couch. We were simply in one another's presence, not talking and only partially focusing on the television show that played in the background.

He started to mumble something and I began the guessing and translating game. What I thought was "I need to shit" actually translated to "How much shit have you been through over the last six months?"

Wow. What a loaded question, I thought. "What made you ask me that?"

"I've been thinking about it for a few weeks now." He knew I had a lot on my plate and I was taking on so much. He saw everything I was doing and in that moment, I appreciated that he noticed.

"A lot," I replied. "I've been through a lot of shit."

For the most part, I am very lucky that Sean's personality has remained the same. He's still caring and comforting and loving. He shows it differently than he did before, but I still feel it. And he's so funny. I've told him multiple times, he's much funnier since his stroke than before.

He got in the bed just the other night, passed gas loud enough for Austin to hear on the other side of the house and said, "It's because of the stroke!" Nice try Sean. Nice try. But I did laugh for a solid five minutes I think. Sometimes, the no filter thing can prompt a lot of laughs too. He's quick witted, honest (to a fault now) and seems to provide me with comedic relief right when I need it. He'll yelp loudly with pain when I'm moving the electric wheelchair making me think I ran over his feet and will start hysterically laughing. He'll compliment me if he likes what I'm wearing, but then also tells me I should maybe wear my hair down instead of up. He might be demanding and want things immediately but he almost always starts it with "please" and tells me "thank you" afterwards.

Stroke brain is a very real thing and it can come in all forms. Someone will be sharing their story about their stroke survivor and I'll think, "do they have a camera in my house? It's like they were talking about us." Other stories will be shared that will make me think how lucky I am to still have Sean be the Sean I've always known at his core. I may just have to answer to "mom," put more salt in his coffee and order a good ol' Chickenburger from Chick-Fil-a for dinner sometimes.

Or maybe I'll just get him a shirt with his motto on it. "It's because of the stroke."

195

PART THREE
WE WILL SURVIVE

Someone once said to me, "I don't know how you do it."

I smiled and replied, "I was never given a choice."

—Ariadna Rios Varemkow

CHAPTER 18

THE TRUTH HURTS

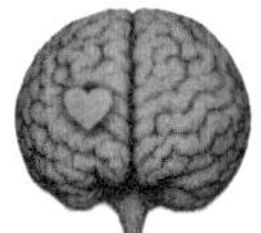

ou can't handle the truth!" That famous line by Jack Nicholson's character from the movie *A Few Good Men* everyone knows whether they've actually sat down and watched the movie or not.

It's a classic line. It's a timeless line. And it's a line that is adamantly true in the life after a stroke, both for the survivor and the caregiver. When I first got confirmation that Sean had a stroke, it literally knocked the wind out of me. Even worse was that the doctors didn't really have an answer for how much this will change his life, only that it WILL change and he WILL be left with deficits. In that moment, I simply couldn't handle the truth. It was like Jack Nicholson was screaming that line straight to my face.

That cold day in January changed our lives forever in an instant. Sean is vigorously relearning how to do everything through all of his therapies. The stroke stripped him from his freedom, his independence, his dignity and his dreams. It stripped me from my dreams as well. All of the things I thought we would do together just may never happen. The ambiguous grief can sometimes be like daggers in my heart that just won't seem to budge or loosen. My boys have been left with a dad that may not be able to throw a baseball with them again or pack up his drum kit to go play a gig on the road. All this may change over time, but right now it is our truth. And that truth hurts.

Accepting the truth is another mountain to climb. I already mentioned that it took me a while to even join a Wives of Stroke Survivor's facebook group, simply because I wasn't ready to accept that I actually was one of those wives. But once I did, I felt heard, acknowledged and accepted. I could share my experiences and realized that other women were going through the same thing as me. It was at least a step in the right direction. It may take a while to accept the different challenges that come with a stroke, but once you do, it makes things a little easier to move on from. Notice I said easier, not easy.

A common scenario I would read about is the fact that the people in your life tend to fall off over time. Everyone is there for you in the beginning when the life changing event happens. The shock of Sean's stroke was a ripple effect through our village of friends and family. We had droves of people, from our present and past, to offer help in the beginning. The amount of love and support was overwhelming and this time I'm using that word in a very good way.

As time goes on, I have noticed that visits are becoming further apart and the phone calls aren't as frequent. Everyone is back to their busy lives with work and their family. And I don't blame them, I'm sure we would even be the same way. I, too, have so much extra responsibility now that I don't have a lot of downtime to sit and "visit" with Sean. It saddens me that his once hour long phone conversations with friends are no longer. Or the last minute invites to the sports bar or golf course simply no longer happen, like he's been taken off the invitation list. Even though all of this is common, and I even got the heads up reading about it, it doesn't make the truth of it all any less hurtful. And if I'm feeling it for Sean, I know he has to feel it too.

When Ricky put on the golf scramble in honor of Sean eight months post stroke, it was one of the best days of the entire year. Those droves of friends and family came back out to support Sean. He was excited to see them and he was greeted the entire day with hugs and comments of how good he looked! Sean couldn't golf that day, but he could drive a golf cart around left-footed to see everyone. He wasn't afraid to talk and mingle. And even though at times, his excitement made him hard to understand, you could still make out enough of what he was saying. That crooked smile of his was on his face the entire day. I'm convinced that it was not only because people that he loved and loved him were there but because he got to feel normal for a day. He got to be one of the guys and hang out with them on a beautiful day and even crack open a cold beer. That normalcy that he got to feel on that one day overshadowed the fact that he was a stroke survivor walking around with a cane and talking a little funny. He was simply just a guy on a golf course, happy to be with his friends.

I miss simply having date nights with Sean. We had finally reached the point in our lives where the boys were older and we could have as many date nights as we wanted. It was great and so freeing for our relationship. The days of scheduling a babysitter weeks in advance were a thing of the past. If we wanted to have a night out, we just went. But now, date night involves packing up the wheelchair, or Sean maybe feeling insecure about using his cane because he's "holding people up" or having to order his food and the server not understanding him. Because of this, we just don't even go out anymore. Something that we used to truly enjoy has become a chore. I want to get to the point where going out to dinner is something we can do together as a couple. I don't necessarily mind the extra effort it takes to go out, but Sean has to work on being okay with it. Until then, the truth is we just don't go out to dinner like most couples do.

A few weeks ago, I was driving to work and my low pressure tire light popped up on my dashboard. I knew it was just a matter of time before that exclamation point lit up on my dashboard. I'm embarrassed to say that I am a fairly intelligent woman in my 40s who has never had to put air in my car's tires. My dad always took care of it when I was younger and then Sean took over when we met. Sean's strengths were my weaknesses and vice versa and anything dealing with cars or house maintenance are my weaknesses. I got home and consulted with my friend, Google. I watched a how-to video on YouTube, dusted off the air compressor in the garage and was determined that I would figure this out. How hard can it really be to put air in tires? I went over to the first tire, cued the video and proceeded to follow the directions, yet instead of air going into the tire, it was slowly seeping out and I was watching my tire slowly deflate in front of my eyes.

Feeling frustrated, I got Sean and he rode his wheelchair out to the garage and proceeded to instruct me on what to do. But the thing was, I was doing what he was telling me yet the tire was still flattening. He muttered, "it's simple." He spun around and went back in the house leaving me with a deflated tire and even more deflated ego. I definitely wasn't proving the fight of "anything a man can do, so can a woman." It was simple to Sean because he's always done these types of things and could probably do them with his eyes closed. Meanwhile, my eyes were filling up with tears from frustration.

The truth was, I was about to have a breakdown over not being able to fill up my tires successfully and Sean not really being able to help me or better yet, just do it himself. And it was because of the stroke. I'll also blame the stroke for the fire department showing up at my front door the day I attempted to change the batteries in our home alarm system. A "simple" task that Sean always handled, but I managed to royally screw up.

Stroke life sucks. I'm not going to sugar coat it. Everyday comes with its own set of challenges. The truth hurts that Sean can't be an equal partner with me. I feel like I'm doing and taking on everything and it can be so much to handle. We can no longer share the responsibilities like we used to. I'm a wife, mom, sister and friend but I'm also a banker, therapist, cook, housekeeper, chauffeur, cheerleader, maintenance (wo)man, consultant, financial advisor, counselor and caregiver, just to name a few. I'm wearing so many hats right now, I could make a killing selling them for the Kentucky Derby next year. I know he sees and hears me struggling, but he's unable to help like he used to before. It's just part of the hand we were dealt and we're both learning to deal with it in our own ways.

Throughout this first year after Sean's stroke, he has only been committed to getting better. Yes, it is overwhelming to take on all my new extra job duties, but his full time job with overtime is simply getting better. It makes it a little easier to take on everything else. Again, easier not easy. He has had his own share of setbacks and one step forward, two steps back moments. He'll accomplish one goal, only to be hit with a new one. Boy, do I know how that feels! It's like your head comes above water, only for someone or something to push it right back down and you're back to gasping for air. For me that something was Medicaid. For Sean, it was being diagnosed with sleep apnea seven months after his stroke.

We went to the respiratory office to be fitted for his new, fancy CPAP machine, a medical device used to treat sleep apnea by delivering pressurized air through a mask while sleeping. Sean didn't want to be there and it was just another thing to add to his long list of stroke related ailments and medications. The respiratory therapist sat a small mirror in front of him and stepped out of the office to gather a collection of masks for Sean to try on. I too had walked out briefly only to come back to see Sean looking at himself, disgusted, in that small mirror. His middle finger was flying high as he looked at his reflection.

"Fuck you!" He was repeating the vulgar phrase to himself over and over while glancing at his reflection and the multitude of CPAP masks that lined the walls behind him.

"Are you talking to yourself?" I was amused at his openness to share his true emotions.

"Yes!" he replied, now equally amused with himself. It was just another thing he would have to deal with because of his stroke. Another hurtful truth about the situation he found his life in. And sometimes it just makes you feel a little bit better to give the stroke a middle finger.

He often asks me in his own words, "am I where I'm supposed to be?" I know he is concerned he is not progressing like he should be. The thing is, everyone is different in their progression after having a stroke or brain injury. That's why doctors can't definitively say what permanent deficits he will or will not have. It truly is unknown. I think as long as you see progression in a forward direction, no matter how minuscule the step is, it's a positive one.

So I tell him, "you're right where you are supposed to be."

Time does ease the pain of the truth and the initial shock of the fact that our family has experienced an event that will change things as we know it. The struggle is real and the road is long and bumpy. Some days are better than others. Some, on the other hand, require you to sit in your car in the garage after returning from work to simply let out a good cry or scream before you walk into the house to deal with a new set of responsibilities. Responsibilities that you didn't ask for, yet they all fall on you. An event that requires you to be strong, yet can make you feel weak. Something that makes you feel so extremely alone, yet the person you love more than anything in the world is right in front of you.

Being a stroke survivor's wife is living with the grief of what could have been, but the hope that things will get better. It's living with pain and hurt of seeing your loved one struggle, but with gratefulness that they are still with you. It is loving yourself and others and realizing that life really is short. Don't spend it being angry, but choose to find the light in a dark situation. Find the new things in this new life that bring happiness and love. This new truth that can hurt so bad can also lead to a lot of pretty great things. You just have to wipe the tears away long enough to find them.

CHAPTER 19
EXTRAS, ECHOES & A GOOD CHECKLIST

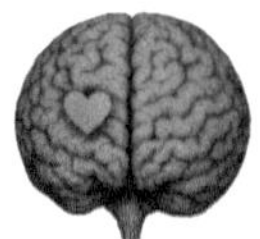

ORGANIZATION EXTRAS

've often been compared to Monica Geller and being a huge *Friends* fan, I take that as a compliment versus an insult, however it was meant to be taken. Monica may not be everyone's cup of tea with her competitive behavior and her obsessiveness about order, control and perfectionism. But she also possesses endearing qualities of being extremely caring, patient and loyal to those most important in her life. I'm proud to be Monica and in dealing with Sean's stroke and everything that goes along with it, I NEEDED to be Monica. Organization and order play a huge part of keeping all the chaos to a minimum, all while preserving my sanity as well.

I really can't fully explain the massive amounts of paperwork that will not just follow you home from the initial hospital stay, but will continue coming in droves from every doctor's appointments and every day the mail carrier fills your mailbox. As an adult, getting mail just isn't as fun as it was as a child. The days of greeting cards filled with ten dollar bills from grandma or receiving your favorite monthly magazine subscription are a thing of the past. Now, it's stifling through stacks of junk mail, ads and bills. Arriving home post-stroke, or any traumatic health event, comes with a lot of no-fun adult mail. Even after almost a year later, the amount has decreased, but I still dread getting the mail everyday.

The Monica in me kicked in when I was already placing daily Amazon orders for the things that Sean would need when we arrived home. I, too, needed my own items to help get me through this new reality. I did not include these items in the Trial and Error chapter because everything I ended up purchasing has been utilized to its fullest extent and I would highly recommend doing something similar to keep everything in order.

First, I purchased a 5-inch three ring binder. If there was a 10-inch one, I would have purchased that. You'll need every bit of the space available. I got a pack of twelve multi-colored folders, tabs and small post-its. Each color folder served a purpose and helped me to keep track of everything and allow me to locate papers in a moment's notice, which I found happened more than I preferred. Examples of folders included medical records, medical bills, work related information, Disability, Medicaid, Trusts, STD/LTD, ABI, TBI, Miscellaneous Stroke Information and Outstanding Items/Things to Do. Pretty much that binder was broken into cate-gories, cross referenced and then color coded…just enough to even impress Monica Geller.

Also color coded was a giant dry erase calendar board that I hung up in the kitchen that everyone could see and access when needed. Each member of the family had their own marker color for the events and appointments related to them. This really became helpful when I was using Mike, Karen and Kathy to help transport to appointments. Everyone could stay on the same page and knew exactly what was going on. The calendar looks like a rainbow every month. Every day is filled with something; Sean's therapy and doctors appointments multiple times a week, Austin's work and drum schedule, my extra curricular events and work schedule,

Landon's college schedule, and when the parents are chauffeuring everyone around. It's chaos, but it's organized chaos and it has been extremely helpful.

MEDICAL BILL EXTRAS

Medical bills started rolling in before we were even fully home. Not much time is wasted before hospitals and doctors are looking to collect their payments. When they first started arriving, I simply opened them up and started a stack on the corner of my work desk. I didn't have time to dedicate to them yet and after all, they'd still be there a day, week or month later. After receiving several of them, I could tell that just my color coded "Bills" folder wasn't going to suffice. I created a spreadsheet to help keep track of everything and to make sure I was being billed correctly based on our insurance plan. I also started receiving the insurance's Explanation of Benefits, or EOBs. Those EOBs were detailed descriptions of EVERYTHING that had been done to Sean and what medical professional was responsible for those procedures. Each line showed the amount that we'd be responsible for paying. When I would receive a bill, I compared the amounts with what was listed on the EOBs. If there was a discrepancy, that led to a phone call to either have it fixed or receive an explanation for the charge in question.

On my spreadsheet, it listed out the payee, what the bill was for, the amount owed, how much of a payment I made and if there was still a balance. Advice from my friends and family regarding medical bills varied from "you don't have to pay medical bills, they'll just end up writing them off" to "don't agree to any payment plan" to "pay everything off immediately." Obviously, everyone's financial situation can be different, so how you choose to handle medical bills can depend on your savings and what you are able to afford immediately. I do not like knowing that I owe someone money. It literally eats me alive. I will pay someone back as soon as I see them or pay off a loan early if possible.

I chose to pay for the "smaller bills" in full, which would be anything under $500. We did have a Health Savings Account with enough funds to cover those. And it allowed me to check them off the list and file in my folder with the hopes to never take them back out again. The bill from the ICU stay was the most expensive bill by far. I did not set up a payment plan, but instead simply sent in random payments on a random schedule. I assumed as long as I was making some payments, I was in the clear. Well, you know what they say about assuming?!

A little over three months later, I walked out to get the mail, as I usually did every day. I was not prepared for what I'd find in the mailbox that day. There were ten plus envelopes all stuffed at max capacity and they were all from a collections agency. I was sick to my stomach, as I opened up each envelope, unfolded the papers and set them in a pile. My eyes started stinging and I tried not to cry as I continued stacking more and more papers together. By the time I was done, I had close to an inch of bills from collections, front and back! I only wish I was exaggerating. I gave myself a few days to process before calling to inquire why I was sent to collections with no warning after only five months post Sean's hospital stay.

Here's what I found out. When you receive a medical bill, you have two options at that point. You can pay the bill in full by the due date or you can set up a payment plan. If you do not do either of those things within three months, even if you are still making some payments, they will send you to collections. At that point, you belong to them. Learn from my mistakes, and just pick one of the two options above. It'll save you the extra stress.

I also found when paying medical bills, that sometimes they will work with you by offering a discount to pay them off in full. I was able to save close to one thousand dollars by doing this with the emergency room bills. If they don't automatically offer it, it's worth inquiring about.

INSURANCE EXTRAS

A little over a month after Sean's ICU stay, I received a letter in the mail from our insurance company claiming that they were denying his last night's stay in the ICU. I freaked out. I was also furious. How could they deny something that I had zero say in? No one ever asked me what I wanted to do. I was just told that he would stay in the ICU until a bed became available at Frazier. I can only imagine how much a night in the ICU would cost out of pocket. I read through the detailed letter and found I was able to appeal the decision. Mind you, I hadn't received a bill (yet), only the denial letter. I immediately began the appeals process. I reached out to his physician's office and requested a letter regarding his need to be in the ICU prior to admission into Frazier Rehab.

We appealed the decision within a week. A month later I received a response stating that there still wasn't enough evidence to keep him in intensive care and once again, we were denied. I was now outraged. I had one more opportunity to appeal, which I did. Thankfully, the nurse practitioner that was writing letters on Sean's behalf was equally outraged and was willing to help me fight this decision. Another letter was sent to argue our side and another denial letter was received. I couldn't comprehend that they thought it would be safe to discharge him from the ICU a day early and do what with him exactly? I definitely couldn't take care of him at that point. He still needed medical attention. Just another flaw in our healthcare system.

After three denial letters for his last night in the ICU, I decided to reach out to the U of L billing department. Several on-holds and transfers later, I got to speak with Chelsea. She looked up our account and it showed a zero balance due. She proceeded to inform me that if and when an insurance company denies coverage (for something that should be covered), they will often request that the patient not be billed for it. So her sweet words of "you have paid all of your bills in full and there are no additional payments required" was music to my ears. Every now and then during this nightmare, you get to have a good call with a positive outcome. So, if you receive a denial letter from insurance, just hold off on getting furious and freaking out. More than likely it will all turn out just fine and you can save your racing heart rate for something else that will probably come up in the meantime.

ECHOES

You will find that you will continue to get the same advice and hear the same comments over and over again. You'll fight between wanting to throat punch someone if you hear it one more time or simply giving into the advice. After all, what will it hurt to at least try? But as a fellow stroke survivor's wife and caregiver, I'm going to echo my advice that I've shared throughout this book. Some echoes are from me giving in to those people who are on "advice repetitiveness" and some are from my own experience that I found to be helpful. In other words, from someone who has been where you are.

- Get yourself at least one homegirl. Or a homeboy, whichever you prefer. They are those people in your life who will not only be BY your side, but pull you FROM the dark side that is very easy to slip into. Lean on them for support and allow them to hold you up when you feel like you're falling.
- Seek out patience, grace and love. You're going to need as much of it as you can possibly get. You need to give this to yourself and to your loved one. No sense in comparing war wounds because you are both going through the trenches in your own terrifying ways. Just be there for one another.

- Accept the help. If someone offers it, take it. Let them bring you dinner, pay a bill, clean a toilet or run some errands. You will be spread thin as is and adjusting to this new reality. No sense in adding more to your plate if someone is offering to take it off your plate instead.
- Find a good therapist. Having a homegirl or homeboy is fantastic and helpful, but you also need a professional to talk too. This is a life changing event that you're going through and it doesn't hurt to get some guidance to balance out the struggles and stresses and simply just help you process everything.
- Love yourself (I prefer this over "Make sure you take care of yourself - you'll hear this a million times. It's one of those throat punching statements. Trust me). However you choose to show yourself love, this is so important to do. I find that when I take the time to love myself, it is literally a reset of my patience. And resetting my patience allows me to care for and be there for Sean in a fuller capacity than I would be if I did not show myself love. This could be as simple as a ten minute walk around the neighborhood so the sun can hit your face or waking up thirty minutes early to sit quietly while enjoying a cup of coffee. It could be meditating, praying or deep breathing. It could be treating yourself to a massage or pedicure, reading a book or going to church. Maybe enjoying a glass of wine or indulging in a piece of your favorite dessert. YOU DESERVE to love yourself. So just do it. And while you're at it, keep the guilt away.
- Allow yourself time to grieve and accept. This could take a lot of time. Even a year into the process, I still have my moments of grieving. It may never go away for all I know, but I shouldn't be made to feel guilty about grieving a life lost or dreams crushed. It's all part of the healing process and are healthy steps to take.

- Find a support group. This could be an in-person group, an online meet up or simply a social media support group. Whatever you find to be the most helpful for you. Talking to people that have been in your shoes and truly know what you are going through and how you feel makes it a little less lonely in the journey.
- Keep hope and faith. It's easy to lose hope when you feel like you've lost so much. I believe there is power in prayer and the moment you give up on yourself, your loved one or God is the moment that hope will be lost too. There's still life to live. It's just going to be different than you thought it would be.
- Continue to dream. If one dream is shattered, make a new one. That's the great thing about dreams. You can have as many as you want and you can make new ones whenever you want to. Consider your dreams like goals. You know you are going to have to work a little bit harder to achieve them, but think of how great it'll be when those dreams come true! Goals and dreams keep you moving forward, and sometimes you need that in order to make one foot move in front of the other.
- Celebrate everything. When you go through something so life changing, simply getting up and surviving the day can be a big feat. This goes for you and your stroke survivor. When things are accomplished, celebrate it. The first time Sean agreed to just go out to eat at a restaurant with me was such a big deal! Normal and mundane for others, but it was huge for Sean. And I got to go on a date with my husband again so it was a win for both of us. But we also celebrated when he was able to squeeze my hand ever so slightly with his right hand. In fact, the smaller things are usually what brings more tears of happiness.
- Don't be afraid to laugh. A lot of this stroke life is serious and sad. It took me a while to give myself permission to laugh or listen to music or enjoy a TV show. But it allowed

such a positive release when I did and I decided to start doing more of it. Plus it helps that Sean is funnier now than before the stroke. And the cute, new country twang that he has developed with his Aphasia makes him even funnier.

A GOOD CHECKLIST

After all the talk I've done about my obsession with checklists, it would only make sense for me to include some for you. I hope you find them helpful and allow you to keep things organized.

AT HOME ITEMS CHECKLIST

This list is composed of items that I purchased along with a list made up by the Kentuckiana Stroke Association. Their items have been compiled from other stroke survivors with items that they found helpful. All items can be purchased on Amazon.

Self-Care/Dressing Gadgets

Several of these items that Sean used were mentioned in Chapter 10.

- Lulex Moccasins for Men House Slippers
- Unenow unisex non slip grip socks with cushion
- AquaDance 7" Premium High Pressure 3-way rainfall combo shower head
- TowelSelections Mens Robe Cotton Terry Cloth Bathrobe
- Elzrghs Commode liners for bedside commode, lavender scented
- Conkote Heavy Absorbency Bed Pad, Washable and Reusable
- LuxStep Shower Mat Bathtub Mat
- aoFit Graduated Compression Socks
- Aircast AirSport Ankle Support Brace

- ClipDifferent Pro 2.0 Electric Nail Clipper with Catcher
- Ableware Press-on One-Handed Nail Clipper
- Luexbox adjustable hair dryer holder stand
- Button Hook and zipper pull one hand buttons aids Button Assist Device
- 27" Dressing Stick
- 35.5" handled shoe horn
- Skechers women's hands free slip ins
- RMS Deluxe Sock Aid
- Kitchen Gadgets - Sean is still learning how to use kitchen gadgets but he has found the rocker knife to be helpful when cutting up meat.
- Keissco Pizza Cutter Stainless Steel knife rocker slicer Knife
- Fanwer Adaptive One-Handed Cutting Board
- Jar Opener for Weak Hands
- Egg Cracker, Automatic Egg Cracking Tool
- Hushee 2 sets adaptive spill proof scoop plates and bowls
- One-handed gadget to secure any item, open jars and bottles
- Ring Pull and Pop Can Opener
- Chef'n EzSqueeze One-Handed Can Opener
- Hamilton Beach Electric Vegetable Chopper
- Arthritis Bottle Opener

Miscellaneous Gadgets

We found these items helpful around the house or while on the go. The grab bars in the shower were and are still a must purchase! As he is standing more and for longer periods of time, I'm looking to purchase even more!

- Proof Latch - Auto Grab Bar Cane Support Aid
- Aqua Silicone Adaptive Aid, Universal Cuff Hand grip assistive device

- Book Page holder - one handed page holder
- Cacoe Phone Lanyard
- 90L Rolling Laundry Basket with wheels
- Kounatsuri Car Handle Assist Handle
- Reyiu Grab Bars for Bathtubs (the first set I bought were great, but second set they changed the design)
- Shower Chair for inside shower with arms and back
- FANhao 2 pa k grab bars for bathtubs

Brain Games and Cognitive Help

- Scrabble Board Game
- The Easy and Relaxing Memory Activity Book for Adults
- Vusign Small Dry Erase Whiteboard
- Amazon Echo Pop
- Stroke Recovery Activity Book - large print: activities and puzzles workbook
- Organization Gadgets
- Maxtek Dry Erase Markers - 6 count colorful magnetic
- Amazon Basics Plastic 3 Hole Punch Folders with 2 pockets, pack of 12

APPLYING FOR ABI CHECKLIST

This information provided by Julie Brennan (the angel) from Caring Moore Homes

WHAT DO I DO NOW THAT SOMEONE HAS HAD A BRAIN INJURY?

For those patients with Medicare, Medicaid and Commercial Insurance - how to apply for Social Security Disability and the Kentucky Medicaid Acquired Brain Injury Waiver that provides needed support services for the patient and family.

There are multiple steps that need to happen before someone can be enrolled in the Kentucky Medicaid Acquired Brain Injury Waiver.

SOCIAL SECURITY DISABILITY

An individual must be found to be disabled under Social Security Disability Guidelines. This application can be initiated by anyone online, by telephone, or in person at their local social security office. https://www.ssa.gov

It is very important that they apply for both Social Security Disability Insurance (SSDI) and Supplemental Security Income (SSI) as Medicaid requires that all potential resources have been applied for.

Little Known Fact: Social Security is required to make an initial determination within 90 days of the date of injury, rather than the date of application. Therefore, applying promptly is advisable, as the benefit start date—and ultimately the financial benefit—are directly influenced by this timeline.

ACQUIRED BRAIN INJURY MEDICAID WAIVER APPLICATION

An individual must select a Case Management company from the approved list. This is who will help the client with all steps to apply for the ABI Waiver. https://www.chfs.ky.gov/agencies/dms/dca/waivers/abiconflictfreecasemanagement.pdf

There are two ABI Waivers available:

Acquired Brain Injury (ABI) waiver: The ABI waiver is for adults with an acquired brain injury who can benefit from intensive rehabilitation services. The services are designed to help participants re-enter the community and function independently.

Acquired Brain Injury Long Term Care (ABI LTC) waiver: The ABI LTC waiver is for adults with an acquired brain injury who have reached a plateau in their rehabilitation level. They require maintenance services to live safely in the community.

MEDICAID APPLICATION CHECKLIST

1. Client's full name and date of birth (applicant, spouse and children)

2. Provide copies of birth certificates for all members of the household

3. Social Security card for all members of the household

4. All insurance cards - including Medicare and Private insurance

5. Value of homestead property (copy of property tax notice)

6. Rental income, proof of cost of taxes, insurance and repairs on the rental property

7. Motor vehicle information (make, model, year of car, estimated value)

8. Life Insurance policies - copy of policy or statement from company showing name of the insured, name of the owner of the insurance, policy number, face value, and cash surrender value.

9. Pre-paid burial policy - goods and services, showing how the policy was funded and proof of irrevocability

10. Bank Statements - 3 full months starting with the most current month for all accounts - including joint accounts and those that are in client's name only and spouse's name only.

11. Copies of certificates of deposits (date issued, amount, owner of CD, last 6 months of activity)

12. Copies of Stocks/Bonds

13. Copy of Trust Funds

14. Proof of Pensions, 401K, IRA, retirement fund, rental income, farm income, etc.

15. Proof of Health Insurance premiums

16. Copy of Power of Attorney / Guardianship Papers

17. Pay Check Stubs - 3 months starting with the most current for client and spouse

18. Current Year Social Security or Railroad Retirement Award Letter

19. Has there been any property sold within the last 5 years?

20. Have you received any accident related payouts as a part of a settlement?

Only if client is married, provide the proof of following living expenses (must be current bill):

- water bill / sewage bill
- gas / electric / heating bill
- trash bill
- telephone bill
- mortgage payment
- Homeowner's insurance

KNOW THE SIGNS OF A STROKE CHECKLIST

The most important checklist, remember BE FAST.

B-Balance - sudden loss of balance, dizziness, headache or loss of
coordination
E-Eyes - sudden blurred vision or trouble seeing in one or
both eyes
F-Face - One sided facial drooping or numbness
A-Arms - Arm or leg weakness, especially if it is on one side of
the body
S-Speech - Sudden trouble speaking, understanding speech or
confusion
T-Time - Time saved is brain saved. 9-1-1 immediately and note the
time the symptoms started

CHAPTER 20

TROK STRONG

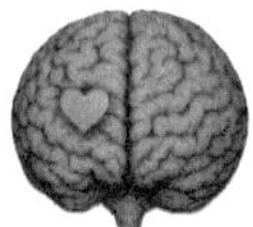

Two days into my daily Sean updates on social media, a friend commented on the status and ended it with *#Trok-Strong*. I loved it. I knew from that point on, it would be our motto for this new stroke life we would be living. Trok, the nickname given to Sean and every other Troklus man, has been a part of him since high school. If he heard "Trok" being yelled, it was a friend calling for him. It was also the name that the ICU nurses shouted out to get him to respond to their pinching and prodding. And the only name that worked to get a response from him. Ironically, the name Trok is also spelled out and sounds phonetically correct in the word Stroke. So I didn't have to put much thought into the title of this book.

Every "Sean Update" I wrote moving forward from day two always ends with the #TrokStrong. It was a trademark of sorts and the catchy phrase became an anthem for Sean's stroke journey. Bracelets were made with the hashtag saying and were given out to visitors when they came up to the hospital. It was to show unity and that we were all fighting alongside him. Once Sean started to become more alert, he got his very own "Trok Strong" bracelet that has yet to be taken off. It is meant to be a reminder to him that he is strong. If he feels like he can't take another step or get his arm up any higher or pronounce a specific word, that bracelet can be a reminder that he can do it and he will do it. In his own time.

T-shirts that were donated to us from Shirley's Way also had the #TrokStrong motto on it. The shirts were red, which is the color for stroke awareness, with a beautiful image of a brain. Except this brain didn't look like our physical brains. It was an artistic image of hands intertwined together to form the shape of a brain. The symbolism spoke so loudly to me in multiple ways. It represented all of the praying hands that were lifting Sean up for the healing of his brain. It also symbolized the healing hands of the multitude of doctors, nurses and therapists that were working together as a team to bring Sean back to us. And it was the representation of our village that were using their comforting hands to hold on to Sean's when they came to visit or to pick me up when I couldn't pick myself up.

Over time, the motto wasn't just for Sean, but for me as well. As Sean would get stronger, I seemed to be getting weaker. I was crying more, bouncing back and forth between home, hospital and work. I was staying so very tired and all of the new responsibilities were piling on. I felt anything but strong. I was in survival mode most days. If I woke up and simply made it through the day to lay my head on the pillow that night, I considered that a win. I was told by others how strong I was, and maybe just getting through the day did make me strong, but I didn't feel that way. Trying to be strong for Sean and the boys, left no strength for myself.

I've always considered myself a strong person, mentally and emotionally. Lord knows, I've been through enough stuff in my life. It definitely shaped and formed me into the woman I am today and in a sense, probably prepared me to take on this big life changing event with Sean. But this stroke journey has required a different kind of strength. It was in me, I just had to find it. And once I did, I did feel strong. I felt really strong.

Sean and I entered into 2026 with a permanent reminder of our newfound strength. We got "Trok Strong" tattoos. He researched and worked on designing the perfect image. Sean wanted to get a tattoo that represented his fight. And his strength. And his grit. And his survival! The image of a stroke survivor ribbon that was worn out and weathered and splintered was perfect. It represented how a stroke tore him down, but he is working hard to piece it all back together. I wanted a tattoo that represented my journey and the path that I continue on with advocating for stroke survivors and their families. The image of an open book — this book — with a flowy stroke survivor ribbon as the book mark. Below each of our tattoos are the words "Trok Strong." We now have something to carry with us forever that represents our strength that we had to find and have to keep to continue moving forward.

It took a good four months before I started to get in a groove with handling things. Tuesdays were my days off from work, but they are far from actual days off. Tuesdays were filled from sun up to sun down with extra doctor's appointments (for myself and Sean), meetings, phone calls and follow-ups. The super woman feeling that I'd get when I would accomplish something that would usually be Sean's duties or finally get a resolution with a medical bill or successfully appeal an insurance denial for a procedure. I felt on top of the world, especially when most of those original calls ended in frustration or tears. I would work so hard to get these things done, for not just Sean, but for myself. I refused to let these things break me and feel weak. I would find that Trok Strong strength to not let it keep me down for long. After all, I am a Troklus.

And the first thing I would do when winning those battles? I'd go straight to Sean and remind him of what a bad ass his wife is and he's so lucky to be married to me! We'd both laugh and he would murmur back while rolling his eyes, "I know!" It was these moments that I knew I could do this and maybe I actually am as strong as others say I am. Sure, I'd still have my moments, but by around month nine post stroke, I really started to get a handle on things. For the first time, I could actually take a deep breath without being fearful of what was going to happen next.

It was month nine where Sean started really hitting a groove too. After being discharged from in-patient rehab at Frazier, he got about a two week break before he was back to work. He had been accepted into the Center for Advanced Neurorehab program (CAN) at Frazier that worked specifically with stroke and brain injury patients, along with spinal cord injuries. They provide comprehensive neurological rehab services that offer innovative treatments using state-of-the-art technologies designed to maximize functional recovery and independence. He was scheduled to attend the CAN program three days per week for seven hour days. During his time there, he had both one-on-one physical, occupational and speech therapies along with group therapies and psychology. They addressed all aspects of rehabilitation - physical, social/interpersonal, cognitive, emotional and life-long wellness. The program was absolutely amazing. The difference they make in people's lives is simply remarkable. They make people stronger.

He was discharged from the CAN program at the end of May after three months with the program. He made huge strides in his recovery. He was on an upward trajectory with his physical therapy and walking so they suggested he continue that throughout the summer while taking a break from OT and speech. So for an additional five months he continued to focus solely on walking. Walking around the gym, up stairs and down stairs, with a cane and without a cane, over obstacles and on treadmills. It was intense but effective. By the end of those five months, he was no longer using the wheelchair at home and was only using a wheelchair when we would have to walk longer distances. Otherwise he was strictly using an aircast or AFO with a cane. Trok Strong.

I have really tried to celebrate the wins and accomplishments, no matter how small. When someone goes through a brain injury of any kind, simple things are actually a really big deal. I wanted to make sure that Sean was celebrated for every milestone that he accomplished. The first time he moved his right leg, we cried tears of joy and then Door Dashed greasy cheeseburgers and thick milkshakes to commemorate the occasion! Peed standing up for the first time (hey, that takes balance)? It was full on cheers and clapping! Saying a full sentence that could be understood the first time around? His face being attacked by kisses! Taking his first steps with no help? More joyful tears and words of affirmation. Man, I was so proud of him that day. Letting the dog outside without me asking? Acknowledging the response and thanking him profusely. They all seem so mundane, yet they are so huge. And I never want Sean to doubt himself or his accomplishments no matter how big or small they are. They deserve to be celebrated and so does he. And I will always be there to cheer him on.

SEAN'S STROKE RECOVERY TIMELINE

1/24/25 - had left brain hemorrhagic stroke

1/24-02/5 - ICU

02/5-2/28 - Frazier Rehabilitation inpatient

2/28 - had feeling in right leg for the first time.

3/6 - had feeling in right arm and bottom of foot for the first time.

3/12-5/30 - CAN program

3/24 - first movement in right leg, bending it at the knee while seated.

3/31 - follow-up MRI appointment. Swelling and bleeding decreases and is no longer shifted over the midline.

4/7 - started feeling "pain" in right arm for the first time

4/14 - started receiving Botox injections in arm and leg to help with tone. - receives it every three months

4/15 - started vision therapy for three months

6/2-10/17 - PT only three days/week

7/25 - overnight in-lab sleep study

8/4 - started companion service through ABI

8/14 - touched his nose for the first time with right hand

8/31 - tiny right finger movements

9/2 - started on CPAP machine

9/3 - started back in OT and speech

9/8 - walked around the kitchen with no cane

9/16 - received his AFO

10/6 - received the Bioness device

9/26-9/27 - first weekend out and about not using the wheelchair at all

10/15 - lifted right arm from lap to on top of the table without assistance

10/16 - walked downstairs in the basement for the first time and back up without assistance (13 steps)

10/17 - last day of PT for the year

10/20 - got up in his truck for the first time

10/25 - out to a nice dinner for our 22nd wedding anniversary - we both deserved that meal!

10/28 - The toilet was running and I couldn't fix it. Sean was able to come over and successfully fix it. I was ecstatic and he was pretty proud.

11/30 - extended all of his fingers on right hand and then purpose-fully closed hand back up. He was able to do that twice on command

1/6/26 - vocational rehab appointment

1/13/26 - driver's evaluation

———

We've all heard the saying that "Laughter is the best medicine." Sean still remains on thirteen medications to this day. Obviously, he needs those medications to help regulate his blood pressure amongst other things, but man, laughter can really be so healing. During this stroke journey, we really experienced the power of laughter a multitude of times, the first time being when he was in Frazier. I had just completed my caregiver training session the day before and we were preparing for the big move home. I mentioned that the training was much harder than I anticipated but I still didn't think I did that bad. Jill and her husband came to visit us at Frazier a few days before discharge to wish us well on our transition.

We sat in a small circle in his big open room and I began telling them about my training session. I was honest about the difficulty of the class, but proud of the "graduation bracelet" I received allowing me to transition Sean around without help. Right in the middle of my story, Sean breaks out into hysterics. I'm talking laughter that comes from the belly as he began imitating and acting out the way I moved him and mocking me of my not-so-graceful transitions.

I wanted to be offended, but the joy that my clumsiness gave him was too good not to join in on. He had us all laughing so hard. And somehow the tears from laughter felt so different running down my cheek than the tears from sadness. And it didn't feel like we were sitting in a hospital room with my stroke survivor husband. It was four friends, who met up for breakfast and shared the best laughs together.

The day that Sean received the electric wheelchair ended up being another laugh-filled evening. What started as a terrified panic of being left alone taking care of Sean all by myself, turned into a family bonding night. We all took turns driving around on Sean's new wheels. Landon and Austin raced around the house, putting it on the turbo speed. We turned all the lights off in the house and got Sean in the chair while he rode around with the headlights on (yes, this thing had actual headlights). It was super creepy (think of the horror movie *Saw*), but was also hysterically funny. Our little family of four that was going through so much change and unknown, got to spend the evening together just laughing. It was exactly what we all needed to face another day.

Before Sean's stroke, we purchased tickets to see the comedian Nate Bargatze who was coming to Louisville in October 2025. We had planned to make a full evening out of it with friends. As the time approached, we began getting concerned about our ticket location, if Sean could go and would we be able to enjoy the evening like we hoped. Sean was fresh off of accepting the fact that he needed a CPAP machine to sleep and I had my latest boxing match with Medicaid. We were stressed to say the least. An hour before showtime, our tickets were able to get switched out for seating to accommodate a wheelchair. We went to dinner before-hand, something that was still a work in progress with Sean, and went to see Nate at the Yum Center in Louisville.

During Nate's one hour comedy set, I managed to cry off every bit of eye make-up that I had on and Sean laughed so hard that I almost missed some of the punch lines. Our abs were aching and our cheeks were hurting by the time we left. That night, there was no stroke and there were no deficits. There were no problems or worries or stresses. We were just a happily married couple going out with friends for dinner and a performance. And we laughed until we couldn't laugh anymore with some of our favorite people and each other.

Laughter is not only the medicine that we all need in life, but I believe it is truly what can help us get through life and its curveballs. It is literally proven to be a real, measurable benefit for both the body and mind. It can reduce stress, lift your mood and improve your perspective on life. It can boost your immunity, relieve tension, be a natural pain relief and improve heart health. And according to Vanderbilt University Medical Center professor Maciej Buchowski, Ph.D., you can lose weight by laughing too! I recently came across an equally powerful saying by Norman Cousins. He states, "Laughter is a powerful antidote for stress, pain and conflict. Nothing works faster or more dependably to bring your mind and body back into balance (than laughter)." In this stroke life that we are living, I am all about finding balance. The bad tends to outweigh the good on many days. But as we continue to heal and recover and move forward, we are starting to find a little more of a balance on the scale of good and bad. One laugh at a time.

We just celebrated Sean's one year "strokeaversary." I found myself dreading the day as it got closer. There was a lot of emotion rising up in me the week prior knowing this day was approaching. Possibly even a little PTSD thinking to myself *this time last year I was on my way home from work to find Sean having a stroke. Will he be okay when I come home today?* And I don't really feel like "celebrate" is the right word to use for the anniversary. Maybe "thankful" is a better word. No, I'm not thankful he had the stroke, but I'm thankful he's still here with us DESPITE the stroke. So instead of celebrating with a fancy dinner out, we simply commemorated the day the best we knew how…with chickenburgers and "white chocolate" milkshakes. And I got to read to Sean the first chapter of this book, all while tears filled his eyes and streamed down my face.

Sean continues to fight and set new goals for himself everyday. He doesn't give up and he keeps going despite the challenges. He is back in speech therapy and physical therapy after taking a break over the holidays. Starting in April 2025, he receives quarterly botox injections in his right arm and leg to help with spasticity and allow for better movement, especially during therapies. In October he was approved through Medicaid to receive the Bioness L300 Foot Drop System. This is a wearable functional electrical stimulation (FES) device designed to treat foot drop and knee instability caused by upper motor neuron injuries, such as stroke. It has been so helpful in his walking and gives him more confidence when out in public settings. He has met with Vocational Rehab, a state-federal program that helps individuals with disabilities prepare for and regain employment. After missing his first Daytona 500 race in 14 years, he is planning to return to that infamous racetrack this year. Something we definitely didn't think would happen last year when we were watching it on a small TV from his oversized Frazier Rehab room. And his biggest goal? To drive and regain his full independence again. He had a driver evaluation in January and with 6 more lessons in a modified vehicle using a left accelerator pedal and knob steering wheel, he could be back on the road by the beginning of March. And doing so in his bright, red F-150 truck.

I found through this first year that you don't always realize how strong you really are and how far you come. Thankfully, I started documenting Sean's progress though pictures and videos from day one. Living in the day to day, you simply just don't realize how far your stroke survivor has truly come. You lose track of time and can lose yourself in the meantime. The impatience will start creeping back in and it's easy to think that everything has just gone stagnant. Nothing feels like it's happening and we're just sitting in place with time standing still. But then I'll pull up a video from just two months ago, and think "you couldn't even lift your arm up and now you can touch your nose!"

Heaven forbid I look back at those pictures from the ICU. Talk about coming a long way. I get so emotional thinking about those moments that I really wasn't sure that Sean would ever lie by me in the bed again. There were days that I thought I would be planning a funeral, not planning out his days. The gift of time is so precious and God decided to give Sean a little more of that and I am eternally grateful to have more time with him. Our life together may look different moving forward but it is far from over.

———

To my fellow stroke survivor wives -

Keep your head up even if the weight on your shoulders is weighing you down. Only the strongest can handle this life.

You are resilient. And even though it may come with a price of giving up your dreams or losing a small part of yourself, there's an even better part of you that maybe you haven't found yet. But it's in there.

You are brave. This life isn't for the weary. We learn to put on a smile and say "I'm ok" even though we are breaking down inside. But we will survive because that's just what we do.

You are loving and compassionate. Your heart is simply making room for a new kind of love that you didn't even know existed. One that cannot even be described to those that have never endured it.

You don't give up. The race is long and the road is bumpy, but you show up anyways. Your endurance and power push through your reality. You show up to care for the one you love but you show up for yourself. Because you need you too.

And you are strong. Your arms are strong from holding the weight, your heart is strong from carrying the grief, and your mind is strong from working harder than you ever thought possible. You are not alone.

Love, Erin, Your sister that you never wanted

As for me, I have come a long way over this year. As I write that message to my fellow stroke survivor wives, I am also writing it to myself. I am a different person than I was just one year ago. Maybe for the worst, but hopefully for the better. The courage and patience I've had throughout this has even shocked me at times. And my love for Sean is greater and stronger now than it was a year ago. And it will be even stronger a year from now. I love his courage, his fight and his strength. And I love his love for me. Together, we can and will survive this. We will run this marathon one step at a time. And the victory of crossing that finish line will be so, so sweet.

We are Trok Strong. I am Trok Strong. You are Stroke Strong.

CONNECT WITH ERIN

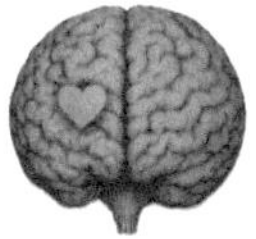

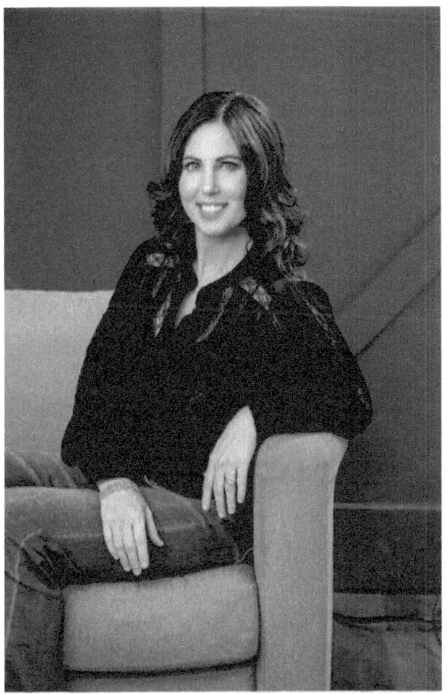

For speaking engagements or podcasts:
strokestrong.erin@gmail.com

facebook.com / StrokeStrongBook
instagram.com / strokestrongbook

The life they knew paused, but their story didn't end.

Sean and Erin met on St. Patrick's Day in 2001 after being introduced by a mutual friend during a fun night out. The connection was instant, and they were married in October 2003, beginning a life together built on love, laughter, and a deep commitment to family. In 2004, they built their first home in a small city outside of Louisville, Kentucky, where they still live today while raising their two sons, Landon and Austin.

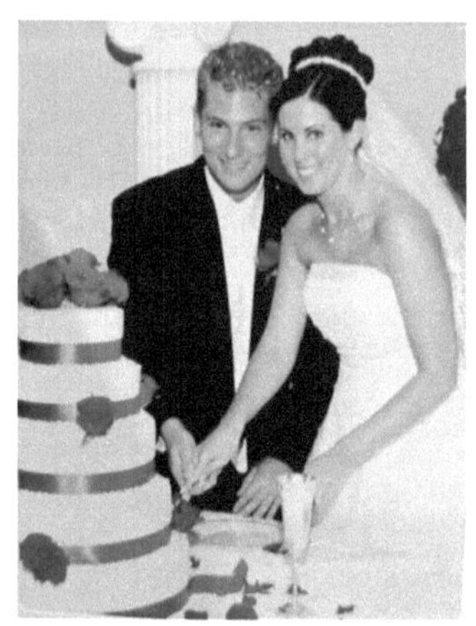

ABOUT ERIN & SEAN

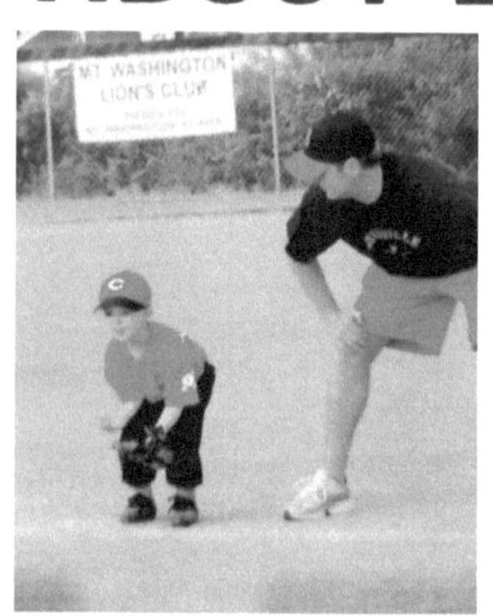

Their family life has always been centered around showing up for one another. Many years were spent at baseball fields, where Sean coached Landon for 12 years while Erin cheered from the sidelines as a proud baseball mom who rarely missed a game. As Austin discovered his passion and talent for drumming, weekends began to include band gigs and live music, adding a new rhythm to family life and countless memories made together.

In 2024, Sean and Erin celebrated their 20th wedding anniversary with a long-awaited trip to Greece—a meaningful time to reconnect and dream about the adventures still ahead.

Just months later, on January 24, 2025, their lives changed suddenly when Sean suffered a massive hemorrhagic stroke at the age of 44.

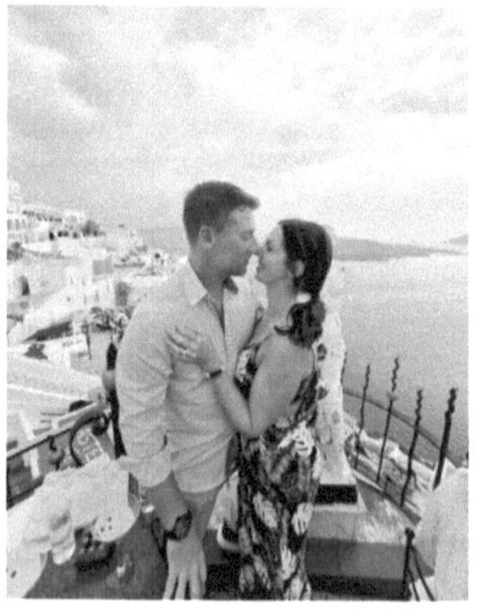

What followed was a year none of them could have imagined. Sean committed himself fully to recovery through intensive therapies, while Erin stepped into the unexpected role of caregiver, advocate, and decision-maker, learning to navigate hospitals, uncertainty, and the emotional weight that comes with loving someone through a medical crisis.

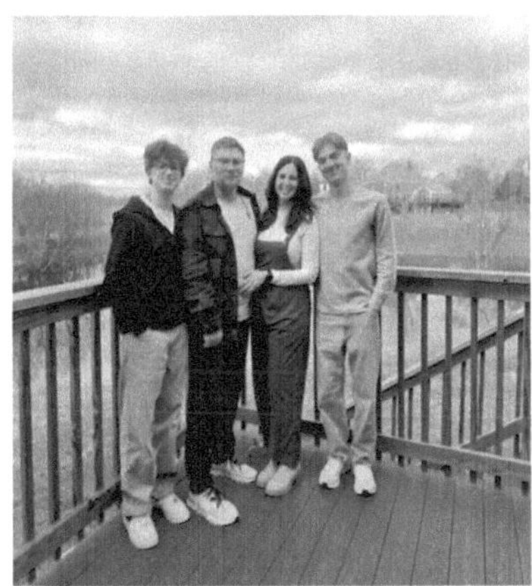

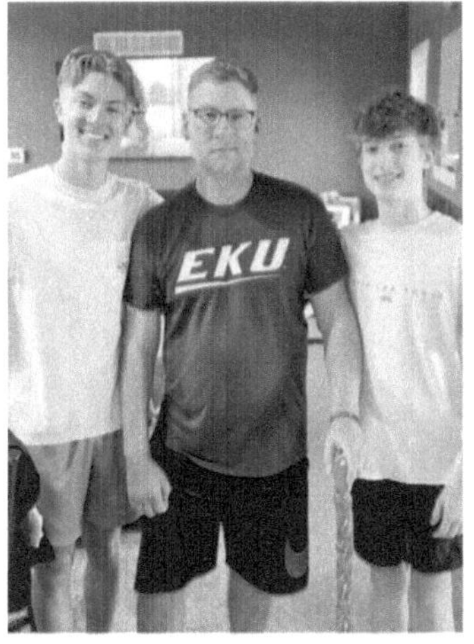

Healing became something they learned together.

With Sean's encouragement, Erin began writing as a way to process their experience and to potentially help others walking a similar path. *Stroke Strong* shares the reality of the first year after stroke through honest storytelling, practical insight, and the hope that families facing the unimaginable might feel seen, supported, and less alone.

Today, Sean and Erin continue moving forward together with deeper gratitude, stronger faith, and a renewed appreciation for the small moments that matter most. Through sharing their story and supporting others on similar journeys, they hope to help families discover their own resilience—and learn what it means to be *stroke strong*, even in the middle of life's hardest chapters.

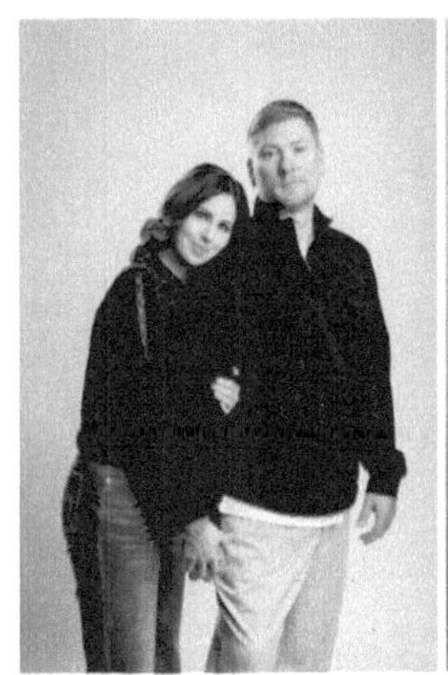

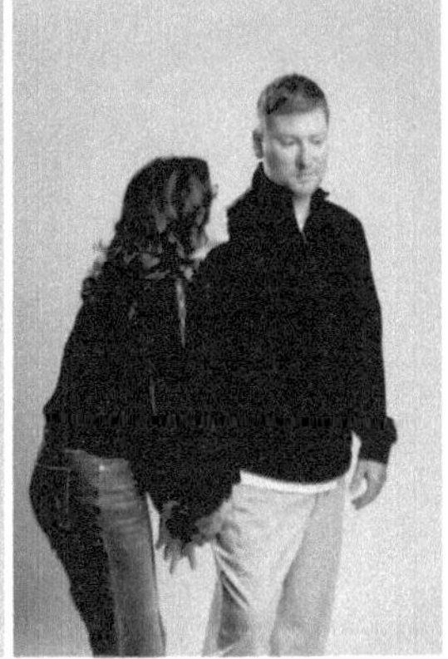

RESOURCES

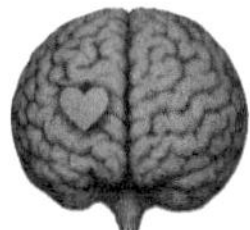

The following organizations and services were available to provide support, guidance, and encouragement throughout Sean and Erin's stroke and recovery journey. Every experience is different, but these resources may help stroke survivors, caregivers, and families find information, connection, and hope along the way.

———

Stroke & Medical Support

U of L Health — University of Louisville Hospital

The primary hospital where Sean received intensive care and specialized stroke treatment during the earliest and most critical stage of recovery. https://uoflhealth.org

Kentuckiana Stroke Association

Provides education, advocacy, and community support for stroke survivors and caregivers throughout the Kentuckiana region. https://www.strokekyin.org/

Emotional Support

Licensed Mental Health Therapists and Counselors

Professional counseling can be an important source of support for caregivers coping with trauma, grief, anxiety, and long-term stress following a medical crisis. Speaking with a trained professional can help families process both immediate challenges and ongoing emotional recovery.

988 Suicide & Crisis Lifeline

Free, confidential support for anyone experiencing mental health challenges or crisis situations. Trained counselors are available 24 hours a day, 7 days a week, offering listening and connection to local resources. Family members and caregivers seeking guidance for a loved one may also reach out for help.

Call or text **988** | Chat online at https://988lifeline.org

Financial & Disability Support

Allsup — Disability Application Assistance

Offers professional assistance with Social Security Disability Insurance (SSDI) applications and appeals, helping families navigate complex paperwork and financial uncertainty during recovery. https://www.allsup.com

Community Support

Shirley's Way

A Kentucky-based nonprofit organization that provided encouragement, publicity through their podcast, a donation to cover publishing costs for this book and #TrokStrong shirts during Sean's recovery journey. https://www.shirleysway.org

School of Rock Louisville

A supportive music school community that encouraged Austin's passion for drumming and provided connection, creativity, and a sense of normalcy for the family during recovery.

School of Rock

School of Rock is a global music education organization that offers performance-based music lessons for children, teens, and adults. Through individual instruction and group band rehearsals, students learn to play instruments, build confidence, and experience the joy of making music together. Many locations also foster strong community connections, providing a supportive environment where families can find encouragement, friendship, and creative expression during both ordinary and challenging times.

To learn more or find a School of Rock location near you, visit: https://www.schoolofrock.com

REFERENCES

The following works are quoted or referenced throughout *Stroke Strong* and offered comfort, perspective, or connection during Sean and Erin's journey.

———

A Few Good Men. Directed by Rob Reiner. Columbia Pictures, 1992.

Bargatze, Nate. *Big Dumb Eyes Tour*. Comedy tour referenced within the text.

Brown, Brené. *Daring Greatly: How the Courage to Be Vulnerable Transforms the Way We Live, Love, Parent, and Lead*. New York: Gotham Books, 2012. https://brene brown.com.

Bruce Almighty. Directed by Tom Shadyac. Universal Pictures, 2003.

Caregiver Action Network. https://www.caregiveraction.org.

Church, Eric. "Like Jesus Does." From *Chief*. EMI Nashville, 2011.

Crazy Town. "Butterfly." From *The Gift of Game*. Columbia Records, 1999.

Friends. Created by David Crane and Marta Kauffman. NBC, 1994–2004.

Freeman, Charlotte. *I Hope You Know*. Thought Catalog Books, 2021. https://www.charlottefreeman.com.

Kent Pateras, Yvonne. Inspirational writings referenced within the text.

Kübler-Ross, Elisabeth. "Five Stages of Grief," concept referenced within the text.

McGowan, Kat. https://www.katmcgowan.com.

McGraw, Tim. "My Best Friend." From *A Place in the Sun*. Curb Records, 1999.

REFERENCES

Stroke Information & Statistics. https://www.strokeinfo.org/stroke-facts-statistics/.

Watkins, Laura. *Something Feels Off: Thriving in Life & Business Beyond a Mental Health Crisis*. Invisible Ink Books, 2025.

Zac Brown Band. "Chicken Fried." From *The Foundation*. Atlantic Records, 2008.

ACKNOWLEDGMENTS

To our parents, Karen, Mike and Kathy - I can never begin to thank you all enough for your unwavering support and love. From the endless loads of laundry, yard maintenance and chauffeur to therapies and practices, I simply could not have survived this first year without you all. It hasn't been an easy year for any of us. You all have experienced your own pain and tears throughout the year, yet never hesitated to still be there for us at a moment's notice. That has never gone unnoticed, even if I didn't thank you in the moment. We are so incredibly lucky to have you all in our lives and as our parents. We love you so very much.

To my boys, Landon and Austin - This year hasn't been easy and it simply isn't fair that you all have had to endure this huge life change. But you did and you did it with courage, strength and resilience. I am so incredibly proud of the young men you have become and how you have handled this life hurdle. You have been there for me when I've needed a shoulder to cry on or the garbage to be taken out. And you've been there for dad while he has been recovering. We are so lucky to have such wonderful, caring boys. I always say, God knew what he was doing when he gave me boys. I thank him every day, but especially this year, that you two are the sons He gave to me.

———

To the medical staff of 5 West at University of Louisville Hospital - I simply can't sing your praises enough. You refused to allow Sean to leave me and there simply aren't words to express my gratitude. You saved his life and you comforted me. You showed him such care and you showed me compassion. You are all blessed with such a gift and you are right in the careers you should be in. Special thanks to "Dr. Queen" and her team. You are miracle workers. To nurses De'Asia, Damien, Eric and Isaac. You treated Sean like a friend. Talking to him like a man, not just a patient. To all of his therapists, especially Ken and my homegirl Sara. Sean may not remember his time in the ICU, but I do, and you all are the ones I remember the most.

To the medical staff on the 7th floor of Frazier Rehab (Room 711 to be exact) - You all gave Sean the motivation to fight. Special thanks to "Dr. Famous" and his team. You deserve every bit of the joy you must feel being a part of giving life back to patients. To Sean's therapy team, Sammie, Megan, Rachel, Cal, Dr. Jensen and Dr. Cheryl. You pushed him to his limits and didn't allow him to give up, but did it with such kindness. To all the nurses and nursing assistants that cared for Sean during our "Temporary Home" stay. Each and every one of you are amazing. To the nurse that spilled his urine after waiting 8+ hours for him to go (you know who you are), you were my favorite. Leaving all of you after our month-long stay, felt like leaving family.

To all of his wonderful Frazier outpatient therapists that he had from month three on - Janet, Maggie, Rosemary, Dr. Amy, Brooke, Suzanne, Christi and Denny. Each and every one of you are playing an intricate role in his recovery and a huge part of bringing back his independence and self worth. No amount of thanks will ever be enough.

To all the social workers Sean has had over this year - You have been there to answer my questions, have breakdowns on and scream at. Every time, you stood there and took it. You have wanted nothing but the best for Sean and our family and your guidance in this journey has been a lifesaver. Keep spreading those wings Sarah, Sara, JoAnn and especially my angel, Julie.

To Sean's companion, Michael - you came into Sean's life at just the right time. Our parents were back to their routine, I had to work and boys were back to school. After two companions quickly coming and going, you came along and were the perfect fit. You gave him the time to accept that he needed a companion and was there when he was ready to get to work. Thank you for talking to him and listening to him. Being patient and kind, but most of all, encouraging him. You were the first person that got him to walk downstairs!

———

To my Homegirls - you got a whole chapter, what more do you want!? How about another THANK YOU?! Thank you for being in my life. Thank you for refusing to let me crumble without you being there to hold me up. Thank you for making sure I ate something and for my hospital care bag. Thank you for loving me and for loving Sean.

To my sister, Kimberly - You've been the single most unwavering person in my life. Not to mention the sweetest and most thoughtful. I can always count on you for anything and I thank God he made us sisters.

To my HR rep, Kelly - I simply could not have made it through the ICU phase without you. You were my voice when I couldn't speak and you were strong when I was too weak to take care of business. I never had to ask you, you simply just did it. Because "you're my people."

To my friend, Ali Williams - thank you for introducing Sean and I all those years ago. You may have missed your calling as a matchmaker, although you're also the only dental hygienist that Sean doesn't hate. Thank you for sitting with me at the hospital for so many days just so I wouldn't feel alone, even if we didn't say much. But when we would talk, you always made me laugh. Sorry you got your hand wet when you picked up a tube off the hospital floor, but you did win the thumb war fight with Sean (silver lining)! You truly are the definition of a lifelong friend. Thank you to you and Erica, too, for making sure I still get out of the house for girls dinners.

To my bro-in-law, Ricky McGuire - the truth is, you drive me completely crazy. That being said, I simply can't imagine life without you in it. You were there for me during one of the worst days of my life and I can't thank you enough. Your usual I-don't-give-a-shit attitude was replaced with nothing but love. Love for me and love for your brother. Thank you for answering my call that day and being the one I could turn to when things turned bad. There's never been a time you haven't been there for the Troklus family when we've needed you.

To Joey and Family - thank you for sharing your time to stay with Sean while in the hospital, so that I could go home just for the night to reset my emotions and take a much needed shower! You became a sounding board for me and gave Sean a little guys' time, which was desperately needed. The #TrokStrong bracelets were a hit too!

To my nephew Michael McGuire and the EKU Sigma Chi Fraternity - you being there for Landon on that horrible day will never be forgotten. Michael, you dropped everything to drive four hours to get Landon and bring him to see Sean. Not because he's your cousin, but because he's your best friend. I cherish the friendship you all have and I know he wouldn't have wanted to make that long car ride with anyone else. To Sigma Chi, you made sure my boy was never alone during the unimaginable four hours he waited to get picked up. And knowing he had his brothers to be there for him when he returned to EKU, made my mom heart so thankful.

To our Trokins crew - Laura, you used to just be my boss, but have become such a valuable friend in my life. I can always depend on you to give me sound advice, drop an F-bomb, a guaranteed laugh and an ear that will listen to every tear and frustration that this year has brought. You and Mike (aka Sean's "best bud") are blessings in our life and I am so thankful for your all's support, encouragement and continued Trokin's Date Nights. It means the world.

To my hype girl, Samantha Perkins - THANK YOU for not closing the door in my face when I told you I wanted to write a book, but oh yeah, I don't read. Even if you were hesitant on the inside, you showed me nothing but care and most of all, you believed in my story and my desire to help others. Your encouragement for me to open up completely was such a humbling experience. My writing sessions with you were also therapy sessions and I healed so much simply because you chose to take a chance on me and this book.

To my Editor, Becky Sasso - You are simply an amazing human being. You embraced my story, like so many others, and my vision for this book, and did it all without taking my voice away. I am sorry you had to edit out so many double spaces, while also creating three paragraphs when I had it as one. You made me believe that I really am a good writer, when I never imagined that writing a book is something I would ever do. It was an honor to work with you during this project and I wouldn't have wanted to do it with anyone else. You are doing amazing things ensuring that women everywhere can speak up and tell their stories. Now, don't you have a cat to go take care of?!

To my massage guests and co-workers at Pure Salon Spa - I've been with some of you for almost 17 years. We have been there for one another during divorces, marriages, babies, death and promotions. We've shared stories and shared secrets. You've also trusted me with your self care. Every one of you were there for me while I was on this stroke journey. You allowed me to cry when I simply couldn't hold back the tears (even if it was in the middle of your massage), but also let me fulfill my job because it was the only thing that felt normal to me. Your love, loyalty, friendship and generosity are unmatched. Each one of you, past and present, have been in my life for a reason.

To our School of Rock Louisville Family, Patrick, Melanie, Doug and the 2025 Show Team Families - Patrick, thank you for the private concert at Frazier that brought just a little normalcy into our very abnormal life. "Chicken Fried" by Zac Brown Band was my favorite. Melanie and Doug, you don't just run a music education school but you run a family. Thank you for allowing Austin to keep his normalcy and continue to stay at SOR. You all are such an important part of his life and our's and you are doing great things with music for our young musicians. To the parents, thank you for the meal train, the anonymous donations to Austin, the grocery trips and for the coffees brought to me in the hospital. Every gesture will be remembered. Rock on!

To Shirley's Way founder, Mike Mulrooney - you are positively touching so many lives in the charity work that you do. Don't let anyone take your light. Thank you for helping so many families suffering through difficult times and thank you for helping my family. Your generosity saved me multiple times. Thank you for believing in my book before even reading it and not hesitating to support the publication of this memoir, simply because it could potentially help so many others.

To all of our extended friends and family - the love and support you've shown Sean and our family is simply overwhelming (the good kind). I have read every text, card and private message that you have sent. Thank you for checking in on me, following his journey and celebrating his victories from near and far. And thank you mostly for all the prayers sent our way. Our prayer warriors have been the best of the best. Love to you all. #TrokStrong

www.ingramcontent.com/pod-product-compliance
Lightning Source LLC
Chambersburg PA
CBHW051313130726
47987CB00004B/1785